A MATTER OF
LIFE AND DEATH

Front cover photo

A 20-year-old Afghan woman, who is pregnant with her third child in three years, is visiting a female elder after suffering abdominal pain and breathing difficulties. She is afraid for her life because she knows how many other women in her village have died during pregnancy and childbirth. They are not allowed to leave to seek medical help and the elders have little to offer apart from some ineffective traditional remedies. There is no modern contraception, early termination, antenatal or safe maternity care.

Cover photo: © Alixandra Fazzina/ NOOR

A MATTER OF LIFE AND DEATH

Women and the New Eugenics

• THE ISSUES
• THE BATTLES
• THE SOLUTIONS

BARBARA ROGERS

Author of *The Domestication of Women*

BROWN
DOG
BOOKS

Published under licence by Brown Dog Books,
7 Green Park Station, Bath BA1 1JB
www.selfpublishingpartnership.co.uk

ISBN printed book: 978-1-78545-244-4
ISBN e-book: 978-1-78545-245-1

Cover design by Kevin Rylands
Internal design by Andrew Easton

Printed and bound in the UK

CONTENTS

INTRODUCTION

To say that family planning and "population" issues are a difficult topic would be an understatement. There is so much known and written about the numbers, and yet the issue of how women can make their lives better and safer through greater control of their own fertility is taboo: no real debate allowed.

You could almost think that since only women can bear children, and this is about women's bodies, that the taboo is stuck in an age of ignorance and silence about sex, women's bodies and childbirth. Yet it is often the supposedly progressive men working in the international sphere who maintain the silence on this, with the quiet complicity of many women. The irony is that these women and men do not hesitate to take full advantage of modern contraception for themselves, and would erupt in rage if there were any attempt to stop them, yet they oppose it for others. Double standards rule.

Is it an exaggeration to say that this is about life and death, especially for the poorest of the poor? This is about births, synonymous with producing a new life - often in dangerous and difficult circumstances. Decisions about whether to have children, and if so when and in what circumstances, are basic life decisions.

It is also about death because of the huge numbers of deaths and injuries to women and their babies from a combination of poverty, inadequate maternity care, poor health and nutrition, and a lack of effective and safe contraception for the prevention or early termination of unwanted pregnancy. It is life and death for people but unfortunately it has become submerged in heated discussions about "population".

"Population" has become a dirty word for many who consider themselves politically aware: "So you're in favour of population control, are you? That would be eugenics then!" These claims are silencing strategies, and they are wrong. But talk of "population" without considering what it really means for individual people feeds into this kind of argument.

It has become a cliché that the personal is political, but it is true. "Population" is personal as well as political. We need to decide which side of the debate to start from: global numbers of people, or individual needs? Many volumes have been written about "population", and the effect of increasing numbers of people on natural resources, the environment and climate change.

Many of these studies, almost all of them written by men, end with a brief reference to family planning: even at their most generous the argument is: let's not examine this in too much detail but perhaps it might be a good idea after all…

I decided that although the numbers are important to keep in mind, this is not the right starting point if we are to be effective in the debate. We should begin with individuals, families and communities, and focus on women since we bear the costs of pregnancy, childbirth and most of the child rearing. Many women have no access to modern means of contraception, and even more have no means of terminating unwanted pregnancies safely and effectively. The result: women and even young girls are being forced to have babies when they are not physically or emotionally ready, with a severe risk of death or permanent injury.

Many babies are also being born into a world where – if they survive – they will suffer from hunger, sickness or disability, with little or no education and poor prospects for the whole of their lives. They may have no job, no land and no means of earning a living. With increasing numbers of children, whole families may be plunged into deepening poverty.

Alongside this there is a worldwide epidemic of dangerous abortions as women try to avoid all this. These often-botched abortions lead to the already inadequate health services being overwhelmed with casualties, while huge numbers of women die from abortions as well as childbirth. In many cases they leave their existing children as orphans whose chances in life are particularly bleak.

The world does indeed face a crisis of numbers. Although high birth rates worldwide are actually declining, the survival of babies and infants is improving much faster. Rapidly growing human numbers are concentrated in the poorest areas of the poorest countries: this is an issue of extreme inequalities, within countries as well as between them. Such areas often have the most fragile environments, which people have no choice but to exploit for short-term survival.

We will never solve the problem by remaining mesmerised by the numbers. We can solve it only by focussing on individual needs and decisions, individual health and welfare, and the forces that are depriving people of their ability to make their own decisions. This book looks at some of the issues, and particularly the organised opposition to family planning and the individuals' control of pregnancy and birth. Our opponents are insisting that there should be more and more children, regardless of the suffering involved or the costs to society.

Nature is cruel: human fertility, left unchecked, produces many more children than we can look after. Pregnancies fail through miscarriages and stillbirths, babies die and women die or become disabled. Control is key: our own ability to control the number and spacing of our pregnancies. This "people's control" is the exact opposite of "population control" by others.

Part 1 of this study reviews why this is a critical issue for women in particular. For men it can be a matter of opinion whether there should be modern contraception, while for women it is truly a matter of life and death. I offer a brief overview of the important projects and programmes being offered now to introduce modern family planning, and some of the innovations that are being introduced.

With the increasing sophistication in the delivery and evaluation of contraception and early terminations of pregnancy, these should be better publicised and made available across more regions and countries.

In Part 2, I examine some of the issues and arguments, including the role of fundamentalism and eugenics, the exaggerated fear of an "ageing society" if our numbers become stable, and the strangely modern evolution of Catholic Church dogma against family planning. I also review the battles being fought on this, from attacks on family planning clinics to battles in the international arena.

Finally, in Part 3, I put forward some new ideas about how to present the issues – as needs rather than rights – and what can be done on the international scene to kick-start a new approach to this crucial issue of economic and social development, and the battle against poverty. This will involve integrating development with health services, and including family planning as an essential element.

Some statistics are inevitable, especially on this topic, but I have kept them to a minimum since the emphasis should be on individual and family needs, and a challenge to the silence that largely surrounds the issue on an international scale. We need to change the debate, and break the silence.

PART ONE: INTRODUCING FAMILY PLANNING

Chapter one

MODERN CONTRACEPTION
and why it matters

The issue of "population" or family planning is surrounded by the dry statistics of demography: abstract numbers and not individual people's lives. It is critical that we understand what really lies behind the topic: the deaths of so many young women who should have their lives before them. Having more children than your health can sustain, or your family can feed and care for, is a tragedy. Dying during pregnancy or childbirth is a terrible reality for many millions of women all over the world. We rarely, if ever, have to confront this loss. But no discussion of "population" can be realistic unless we do.

I have chosen a few of the descriptions from Badakshan, Afghanistan by the photographer Alixandra Fazzina, who took the image on the front cover of a widower and orphan child following the death of yet another woman in childbirth. This is inequality and poverty at its most extreme.

Gulzaman, a widower, sits with his orphaned daughter. Her mother Zakria died four years ago during childbirth and spent seven days in terrible pain, moaning and crying, before she died. Gulzaman prayed to keep her alive but there was no medical help. The little girl, who witnessed all of this, became withdrawn and cried all the time. She has now been sent away to live with her grandparents and will probably be married soon and have to face the same trauma herself. Her father has now taken another wife.

Baguma tries to make the two-and-a-half-hour journey on foot from her village to the nearest clinic, suffering from severe pain and bleeding. She never makes it but has to give birth behind some rocks, then turns back with the new-born baby still attached to her, wrapped in a blood-soaked burka. Since then no woman in her village dares to seek outside help in case this happens to them.

Sangimo lies on the operating table at Faizabad Maternity Hospital having arrived in great pain, with heavy bleeding and struggling to breathe, following a 12-hour journey by jeep across mountain roads. She is four months pregnant and has already had four miscarriages. Her husband has sold all their land to get her to the hospital. His first wife died during childbirth.

Zebanisa struggles to care for her orphaned granddaughter Fahima in one room in Khourdakon village. Her mother was 27 when she died in great pain during childbirth. "There was nothing I could do – I just had to stand by." They managed to find transport across the mountains for the seven-hour journey to Faizabad Hospital, but by the time they got there it was too late to save her life. Fahima's father has rejected the child, as is often the case when the mother dies in this way. Zebanisa, although in deep shock, was the only person who would take her. She and her granddaughter have no means of support and can survive only through help from her neighbours, who are themselves struggling.

A traditional birth attendant is holding her empty toolkit, in which she should have basic equipment to help with childbirth. Until recently, she used flints for cutting and piles of earth for soaking up the blood. Now, following a training course seven years ago, she wants to use plastic gloves and sheeting, and sterilised razors and needles, but these are often unavailable. "I always reassure the women in delivery, but there is nothing I can really do," she says.

From Nepal there is another report of too-frequent, unsupported and dangerous pregnancy as a threat to the lives of women. An account from the poor area of Accham by film-maker Subina Shrestha – who was herself pregnant at the time – gives some sense of the fear that many women have:

"Laxmi [a nurse] had tales of women dying while giving birth. She talked about women who begged to be saved but their family refused to take them to a hospital, and of women whose vaginas were hacked by village 'healers' after their baby died inside them. No wonder Basanti was so keen to have us around. It meant that we would not let her die.

"Tales of women suffering in Accham could make any sane person's blood boil. Even if women survive one childbirth, they might die in the next one. If they have daughters, they are obliged to keep trying until they have several sons. Those who live through it all might have a prolapsed uterus. When I think of the fate of 13-year-old Sunita, it breaks my heart. Accham is like a black hole where women's dignity is destroyed. Even before the filming ended, all I wanted was to get out of there."

Women's lives and deaths

We can understand a little of what it is like for a few women in one community, but the sheer scale of this is almost beyond our imagination. Random and uncontrollable pregnancies are a huge threat not only to women's lives and health, but also to the welfare of whole families and communities. Every year in developing countries women have about 89 million unintended pregnancies, almost half of them (43%) being unplanned. Of these, women's fear of pregnancy leads to about half being ended by abortion, most of these desperate and dangerous, and leading to widespread deaths and severe disability. Globally, the numbers of these deaths far exceed most epidemics. In 2014, which saw high death rates from the Ebola epidemic, there were four times as many deaths from abortion.

There are an estimated 48 million abortions, 10 million miscarriages and one million babies born dead every year. It is estimated that 214 million women are unable to get family planning when they need it. The figures would be impossible to ignore if this was any other international issue. Planning for children, and the births and deaths that arise from women being unable to get modern contraception, are the biggest single issue for women worldwide. It is also very much an issue of poverty and inequality. The rate of deaths of women in childbirth in the least developed countries is 436 per 100,000 births, compared with just 12 in developed countries. In other words, deaths are 36 times higher in the poorest areas than the richest ones.

Unintended pregnancy is closely linked with the women's issues that are now on the international agenda. They include forced marriage, rape, female genital mutilation (FGM), sexual harassment and domestic violence, together with discrimination in education and jobs, and exclusion from the modern economy. It is particularly acute for girls who are married off as children, sometimes even before puberty: we are talking here of child sexual abuse or rape, being forced to work for the husband and his family without pay, and being made pregnant before the young girl's body is ready and when childbirth is particularly dangerous, both for the girl and for the baby. These are often treated as single issues but for the woman concerned it is all one: her whole life. Sex and pregnancy at too young an age, and births that are too closely spaced, impose a serious burden on women's health, and that of the babies.

Most of the women with an unmet need for contraceptives live in 69 of the poorest countries on earth. For many, there is no family planning service of any kind. There may be no health services at all, or some kind of provision from a Catholic or Islamist clinic, which excludes contraception and early terminations altogether. The UN Fund for Population (UNFPA) reports that "the unmet need for family planning in developing countries is generally greatest among women in the poorest 20% of households". This particularly applies if they are less-educated and living in rural areas, and is even more extreme for adolescent girls, who are forced into sex with older men and have little power in the relationship, in some cases being repeatedly raped by their husband or partners. The UNFPA adds that inequality in family planning access intensifies the divisions in society: closing the gulf between women in income, education and employment will largely depend on enabling all women and girls to meet their reproductive needs. "Inequalities in sexual and reproductive health and rights have implications that run from individuals to entire nations … A poor, uneducated woman in a rural area who cannot make choices about pregnancy will be unlikely to gain an education or join the paid labour force. As a result, she will probably remain trapped in poverty and marginalization."

The level of unmet needs closely mirrors levels of poverty. Just 2% of women in France have an unmet need, while in Samoa it is 46%. Africa is a particular area of need: almost half of the 44 countries with the required data have unmet need levels of over

20% of all women of reproductive age who are married or in a union. For over a quarter of these countries this is over 30%. Even where some modern contraception is available (especially with condom-only programmes to combat HIV/AIDS) women and girls may not have the men's agreement to use it. A limited range of choices in many areas means that women and couples may not be able to get the most effective method for them.

Worldwide, only 57% of women aged 15-49 who are married or in a union were using modern contraception in 2016, and this figure falls to only 35% in the least developed countries. Inequalities exist between and within countries, with the greatest need among the poorest people, young unmarried women, poorer and less-educated women, and those in rural areas. This is also a feature of conflict zones and among refugees and migrants: South Sudan, for example, has one of the highest rates of maternal mortality in the world, together with one of the highest fertility rates: almost five children on average for each woman. The highest levels of need are in Sub-Saharan Africa and in Southern Asia, especially India, Indonesia, Pakistan and the Philippines.

Maternal mortality closely matches the levels of **poverty** within countries. For mothers as well as for their infants, the risk of dying during or shortly after birth is 20–50% higher for the poorest fifth of households than for the richest fifth. In Chad, for example, only 1% of the poorest women are attended by skilled health personnel during delivery, compared with 48% of the wealthiest women in that country.

A woman's lifetime risk of maternal death – the probability that a 15-year-old woman will eventually die from a maternal cause – is 1 in 160 in developing countries, compared to 1 in 3,700 in developed countries. The combination of poor general health and nutrition, pregnancies too young or too closely spaced, the lack of skilled health personnel to help with the birth and dangerous abortions are all factors. For girls under 15 years old, complications of pregnancy and childbirth are the leading cause of death. High levels of child marriage in some countries is contributing to this mortality, and so is the abuse and trafficking of girls. They simply do not have the information or the means to start protecting themselves, since there is very little sex-and-relationships education for young people. At the same time, worldwide distribution of pornography portrays girls and women as targets of sexual use by men, and rarely even mentions protection against involuntary pregnancy.

What is reproductive health?

Good sexual and reproductive health, as defined by the UN Fund for Population (UNFPA), is a state of complete physical, mental and social wellbeing in all matters relating to the reproductive system. It means that people are able to have a satisfying and safe sex life, the capability to reproduce, and the freedom to decide whether, when, and how often to have a child. To maintain one's sexual and reproductive health, women and men need access to accurate information and the safe, effective, affordable and acceptable contraception method of their choice. They must be informed and empowered to protect themselves from sexually transmitted infections. And when they decide to have children, women must have access to services that can help them have a fit pregnancy, safe delivery and a healthy baby. This is the ideal, and it is largely achievable by most people in the richer countries.

Improving maternal health was one of the eight Millennium Development Goals (MDGs) adopted by the international community in 2000. Under MDG5, countries committed themselves to reducing maternal mortality by 75% between 1990 and 2015. This target has not been met: the reduction in that time, although a great achievement, is a long way short of the target at just 43%. Clearly, the failure to provide safe and effective contraception, alongside poor health systems and inadequate obstetric services, has been a major factor in this failure.

The new Sustainable Development Goals (SDGs) have a further target of reducing worldwide maternal deaths from 239 per 100,000 to under 70, with no country having more than double that. Comparing this with the rate in more developed countries of just 12, this should be the very least that can be expected. Unfortunately, the target is seen as very difficult to achieve as long as there is so little funding for programmes to improve family planning services within a basic health structure.

In 2015, the World Health Organisation estimates, 830 women were dying from pregnancy- or childbirth-related complications around the world every single day. And for every woman who dies, 20 or 30 more encounter health complications with serious or long-lasting consequences. One of the most common is fistula, caused by the baby being in the wrong position or too large for birth which leads to obstructed labour. Adolescent girls are especially vulnerable to this. A good health service would proceed to a caesarean section to enable a safe birth in this situation. Without that, the woman is forced to go through days of agonising pain and exhaustion. Eventually the foetus suffocates. The unrelenting pressure on the soft tissue of the mother's womb greatly reduces the flow of blood to the soft tissues surrounding the vagina, bladder and rectum. The injured soft tissue can die and creates a hole (fistula) through to the bladder or rectum, which will cause her to become incontinent, leaking urine or faeces through her vagina for the rest of her life. Not only is this horrible for the woman if it is left untreated but it can lead to her being shunned, thrown out of her family and excluded from her community.

For each woman who dies or is incapacitated, there is usually a family – often with several children – that is plunged into disruption, hunger and intense poverty. The risk to health is illustrated by the numbers of women becoming pregnant again too soon after giving birth, endangering their own health and that of their babies. While more than 92% of mothers do not want to get pregnant again soon after childbirth, 61% of postpartum women in low- and middle-income countries are not using family planning methods. At least half of these women give birth again within an interval that is seen as unsafe. Even when a mother is using whatever contraceptives she can get, they may not be the safest or most effective methods.

If all unplanned pregnancies could be avoided, this would provide a huge boost to women's health and survival rates. It would also permit a much higher proportion of babies to be born healthy, with a better chance of good nutrition and able to move out of poverty. The World Health Organisation reports: "Maternal health and newborn health are closely linked. Almost three million newborn babies die every year."

No place for pessimism

It is often argued that attempts to provide contraception are resisted by poor people, who are slow to accept what is offered. Nothing could be further from the truth: where real choice is provided, there is strong demand. The range of effective choices in contraception has greatly improved in recent years, delivery channels have become better, and contraceptives are safer and more effective than ever (although further research and development are still needed). Several developing countries have had very successful government programmes providing opportunities for real choice, which has resulted in much reduced maternal and child mortality and a reduction in numbers of births to replacement level, similar to many developed countries. The list of those making this commitment is not what you might expect. They include low-income countries like Bangladesh, Bhutan, Lesotho and Rwanda as well as medium-income countries like Cambodia, Iran and Thailand.

Worldwide, although there is much still to be done, there has been great progress over the last few decades. Compared to 1970, when only 36% of married or cohabiting women between 15 and 49 were using any kind of contraception – modern or traditional – that figure has now risen to 64% in 2015. Africa as a whole has moved from 8.2% to a still very low 33.4%. Many of these were not using the safest or most effective methods in 2015, and this needs to be addressed, but the change is remarkable. It still leaves many other countries lagging behind, however.

One thing that would accelerate the rate of change would be a full understanding of the economic benefits of modern contraceptive delivery. Not enough work has been done so far to quantify the return on investment here. However there are already some findings of greatly improved health and welfare, together with better household incomes. A study by the Population Reference Bureau in Bangladesh in 2009 found that long-term investment in integrated family planning and child health services in certain areas produced better health and wellbeing than those in a similar comparison area. A typical woman of 38 in the service area had one fewer children, while her body mass index (BMI) rose above the level of risk from under-nutrition and her daughters also had a healthier BMI. The family was more likely to have its own source of clean water, the children were more likely to be vaccinated against crippling diseases, and the family as a whole had more money.

Another very useful review has been carried out by the service agency Marie Stopes International, which has outreach programmes in some of the poorest regions in the world. They estimate, based on their own experience and using publicly available data, that in a typical poor and fragile country, around a third of the women want to limit pregnancies but are unable to do so. If just 5% of these women are given access to modern contraception, the effect on national welfare would be substantial. GDP per capita for the whole population would increase by US$1,700. Completion rates for girls in primary school would rise from 69.9% to 73.3%. There would be an increase in the Gender Equality Index for that country of 2.5 percentage points. Reliance on foreign aid would fall from 32% to 29%, and there would be a decline in its ranking on the Fragile State Index from 91 to 87, moving it out of the "Alert" category. Clearly, if the investment were more substantial than that, the effects would be even more positive. We need more such analysis to make the financial case for contraception and safe abortion. Many decision-makers may be indifferent to the case in terms of women's and families' welfare, but money talks. If it works, do it.

Another set of calculations has been offered by the World Bank with its Global Financing Initiative for health, which aims to introduce cost-effective integrated health care, especially for women and children. They estimate that it would cost just $25 per woman per year to provide integrated health care to women and newborn babies, including family planning, prevention of young teenage pregnancies, ante-natal and obstetric care, prevention and treatment for HIV and sexually transmitted infections, and nutrition support and care for the babies. The benefits would be "almost incalculable". These would include prevention of 52 million unintended pregnancies, 14.9 million dangerous abortions, 194,000 deaths of women, 2.2 million deaths of babies, and 121,000 HIV infections among newborns. They also calculate that poverty, with the stunting of foetal and children's growth, leads to a 26% reduction in their income as adults. This is a serious brake also on national GDP per capita, where stunting alone is estimated to reduce national GDP by an average of 6%, rising to 8% in South Asia and sub-Saharan Africa.

Environmental effects

Human numbers have been increasing exponentially within the lifetime of many of us. In 1950 the global human population was around 2 billion and by October 2011 it had reached 7 billion. By 2017 it was estimated at 7.55 billion people. This is currently increasing at a rate of 1.2% a year and is projected to reach 9.6 billion in 2050, and 10.9 billion by the end of the century, according to the medium variant of the latest UN population projections. This figure assumes an increase in people's access to family planning services; without that the growth could be much faster.

Almost all of the additional 3.7 billion people expected between now and 2100 would be in developing countries, increasing from 5.9 billion in 2013 to 9.6 billion in 2100. In some of the least developed countries, the human population could triple if nothing is done about this issue. Such increases among the poorest populations force people to encroach on fragile ecosystems just to try and survive. The result: destruction and burning of forests, depletion of soil quality and a loss of soil cover through wind and water erosion, expanding deserts, reduction of rivers, lakes and underground water sources, pollution of soils, water and air, falls in fish stocks, loss of pollinators, and the extinction of many plant and animal species as well as the natural ecosystems on which we all depend. There is also an increasing death toll where people are affected by conflicts, become refugees or migrate, often to cities and coastal areas that are vulnerable to landslides and flooding.

The United Nations' Intergovernmental Report on Climate Change, in its Fifth Assessment Report of 2014, identified changes in the human population as factors that exacerbate climate change vulnerability: "Human interference with the climate system is occurring, and climate change poses risks for human and natural systems... Although population growth rates and total population size do not alone determine emissions, population size is an important factor.

One study showed that CO2 emissions could be lower by 30% by 2100 if access to contraception was provided to those women expressing a need for it. Providing the unmet need for contraceptive services in areas such as the Sahel region of Africa that has both high fertility and high vulnerability to climate change can potentially significantly reduce human suffering as climate change proceeds." The report also notes that population increase imposes pressures on water and food availability, and the viability of many cities and coastal communities.

The Low Elevation Coastal Zone (LECZ) constitutes 2% of the world's land area but contains 10% of the world's population (600 million) and 13% of the urban population (360 million) based on year 2000 estimates. About 65% of the world's cities with populations of over 5 million are located in the LECZ and are particularly vulnerable to flooding as sea levels rise.

Security, too, is a concern. In November 2014, the US Department of Defense released the *Climate Change Adaptation*

Roadmap, which predicted more conflicts, forced migration and wars – all consequences partly of increased population numbers and competition for resources. The statement describes climate change as a "threat multiplier" which "will intensify the challenges of global instability, hunger, poverty and conflict. They will likely lead to food and water shortages, pandemic disease, disputes over refugees, resources and destruction by natural disasters in regions across the globe."

Consequences

Without reproductive health, especially modern contraception, efforts to promote health and wellbeing will not work. In particular, the health of women and children, and their whole families, are likely to deteriorate.

According to the latest estimates by the respected Guttmacher Institute, current levels of contraception are preventing the deaths of 100,000 women and 1.8 million newborn babies every year. They are avoiding 144 million abortions, including 38 million illegal and dangerous ones, and 25 million miscarriages. Fulfilling the unmet need for modern contraception in developing countries would, each year, save the lives of another 70,000 women and half a million babies; and avoid 24 million abortions and 6 million miscarriages. If we were talking about an epidemic of disease on this scale, it would be classed as an international scandal and there would be a huge mobilisation of resources to combat it.

It has been estimated that achieving universal access to sexual and reproductive health services by 2030, and eliminating unmet need for modern contraception by 2040, would deliver $120 of social and economic benefits for every $1 invested. Yet since the mid-to-late 1990s, donor assistance dedicated specifically to family planning has decreased dramatically in absolute terms. There has been some increase in donor support more recently, but not enough even to make up this shortfall. There is a huge need for more money. According to the Guttmacher Institute, fulfilling unmet need for modern contraception in developing countries would require an estimated doubling of current global investments from the current US$ 4.1 billion to US$9.4 billion annually.

One of the most constructive approaches to the issue of reproductive choice is as a health issue, with a focus of concern for the individual woman, her partner and their children. Although we have to be aware of the numbers, this is not a numbers game. Trying to tackle the issue in this way (books with titles like "Population Bomb", "Full House" or "Peoplequake") can play into the hands of those who want to portray us as wanting "population control" by outsiders, rather than our real objective of wanting control to be in the hands of the people concerned. A focus on numbers also caters to the obsessions of sectarians who want to increase their own group's population at the expense of others – a key element in so many sectarian conflicts. This is the subject of Part Two of this book.

Seen from the perspective of individual welfare, the task is to provide reproductive health and choices in health programmes – and to improve those programmes overall. Development economists are very much to blame here: they attach little or no monetary value to health, instead focusing on paid work and commercial outputs (and also ignoring the huge amounts of unpaid work in any economy).

In many poor areas, there is a medical and health system that specifically excludes family planning. The networks of Catholic clinics and hospitals are forbidden to offer any choices apart from complete abstinence from sex or the unreliable "rhythm method" of timed abstinence. It would be hard perhaps to argue that the presence of these exclusive health facilities drives out a more comprehensive and valuable health service that also offers contraceptive choices, though there may be an element of that. I will argue that governments should consider taking over such health facilities as part of an official programme. Failing that, they should aim to offer a stand-alone family planning service with equal reach into the poorer communities, and they should insist that Catholic clinics and hospitals should refer their patients there as appropriate. It is not the most efficient approach, but it may be the only practical one. The same issues apply to the health services offered by some hard-line Islamist groups, to poor people in areas where there are no other medical services, which also provide a base for consolidating support for the extremists among the local community.

International, national, local and non-governmental bodies should be challenged to accept reproductive health, alongside other health services, as a key element in any true development programme. It is very striking that many otherwise admirable aid agencies have decided to exclude reproductive health and choices from their programmes. I have found that among British agencies, for example Oxfam and Save the Children, currently do little or nothing for reproductive health. An Oxfam representative defended their position by claiming that "others" will provide this service. In far too many areas in which they operate, that means no help at all. This needs to be reviewed as a matter of urgency.

It is very sad also that most of the specialised agencies of the United Nations, including the World Health Organisation (WHO) and the Children's Fund (Unicef) are not providing reproductive health support as an integral part of their work, for reasons we will explore later. Their line, when questioned, is that this is the job only of the UN Fund for Population (UNFPA), who work alongside them in some areas. However, UNFPA's budget is very small compared to many of the other health-related agencies, and it also has other activities such as census management, which take some of the already limited funds. If real progress is to be made, all relevant agencies must incorporate choice about family size into their programmes, and include it in their budgets.

At the time of writing there is a crisis in the funding of family planning programmes, and particularly the continuing supply of commodities. Christian Saunders of the UN Population Fund estimates that for every $1 million shortfall in contraceptive commodity provision, there will be 360,000 unintended pregnancies of which 150,000 will lead to induced abortions; there will be 800 additional deaths of the mothers, 11,000 deaths of the infants and an extra 14,000 deaths of children under 5. These are sobering figures. For the women and children involved, the reality is catastrophic.

Resources

Unpublished reports from Alixandra Fazzina from the website of Noor Images.

Subina Shrestha, "Birth in Nepal," Al Jazeera *Witness*, 13 July 2012.

UNFPA, *The State of World Population 2017*. All other figures are from Unicef, WHO, the Guttmacher Institute and UNFPA.

"Underuse of modern methods of contraception: underlying causes and consequent undesired pregnancies in 35 low- and middle-income countries," *Human Reproduction* (2015) 30 (4), Oxford University, UK.

United Nations, Department of Economic and Social Affairs, Population Division (2014), *World Contraceptive Use 2016*.

United Nations, *Millennium Development Goals Gender chart*, 2015.

WHO, Unicef, UNFPA, World Bank and United Nations, *Trends in Maternal Mortality 1990 to 2013, WHO*, May 2014.

Rachel Winnik Yavinsky and others, *The Impact of Population, Health, and Environment Projects: A Synthesis of the Evidence*, Working paper 2015, The Evidence Project, Population Council, Washington DC.

Newman, K. and Fisher, S. (2010) *Population Dynamics and Climate Change: A PSN Briefing Paper*. Population and Sustainability

Network. Available at: *http://populationandsustainability.org/wp-content/uploads/2014/10/Population-and-Climate-Change-Briefing-Sheet.pdf*

Singh, S., Darroch, J.E. and Ashford, L.S. (2014) *Adding It Up: The Costs and Benefits of Investing in Sexual and Reproductive Health 2014*. New York: Guttmacher Institute and United Nations Population Fund.

Copenhagen Consensus Center (2014) *Benefits and Costs of the Population and Demography Targets for the Post-2015 Development Agenda*.

Population Reference Bureau paper 2009, *Family Planning and Economic Well-Being: New Evidence From Bangladesh, available from their website*.

Marie Stopes International, *Time to Invest: The case for contraception as an investment for the future,* published on their website, 2016.

Christian Saunders, UN Population Fund, "Differential Pricing: UNFPA's Experience with Contraceptives," on the UNFPA website.

World Bank Group, *The Global Financing Facility: Country-Powered Investments for Every Woman, Every Child*, 2016.

Chapter two

WHAT WORKS
Local knowledge, international expertise

It is sad how little is known in the wider development community about the success stories of family planning. Is this the best-kept secret on the international scene? This is not the place for a comprehensive overview, but my case for a new approach would not be complete without some reference to the work that has been done, and continues to be done, to enable people to decide whether and when to have a baby and to allow women to stay healthy and have healthy children. I have selected a few examples to illustrate the wide variety of successful approaches that have been developed.

Methods

First, we should quickly review what contraceptive methods are available. In the popular view there is only the hormonal birth control pill for women, or condoms for men, supplemented by sterilisation for women (by tubal ligation) or men (through vasectomy). Otherwise there would only be the hit-and-miss rhythm method of abstaining from sex altogether during a woman's most fertile phase. Germaine Greer's *Sex and* Destiny, for example, shows an extreme lack of understanding of the available methods at the time it was written. But the science and rigorous testing of new contraceptives has produced a wide variety of methods, which go way beyond this.

Perhaps the most significant are the LARCs (long-acting reversible contraceptives). They can be delivered by injection, which previously required a trained health worker. In 2016 it was made much easier with the Sayana Press, a pre-filled, single-dose syringe and needle in an all-in-one package, which can only be used once, so that no infection can occur. It is very easy to administer or even to self-inject as is done with insulin injections by diabetics. This important innovation is the result of three decades' work involving dozens of cross-sector partners, including pharmaceutical companies and a variety of governmental and private aid donors.

Other LARCs are implants under the skin, which can last for up to five years but can be removed at any time to restore the woman's fertility. There is also a variety of intra-uterine devices (IUDs) which are inserted into a woman's uterus. These are also long acting and easily removed.

The US National Institutes of Health list a wide range of other types of contraception licensed for use there. They start with barrier methods: diaphragms, cervical caps, female as well as male condoms, and contraceptive sponges, which can all be used on their own or with spermicidal gels or creams. Hormonal methods include patches, vaginal rings, implantable rods, and pills that can be progestogen-only or combined with oestrogen. Intra-uterine devices are available as copper or hormonal IUDs. A variety of shapes, sizes, formulas and makes are often available for each category. In addition, emergency contraception after unprotected sex includes inserting an IUD or taking hormonal "morning after" pills, up to five days after unprotected sex. Sterilisation now includes non-surgical implants for women, which seal the fallopian tubes within around three months, as well as surgical tubal ligation for women or the much simpler vasectomy for men. Work has even been done on the rhythm method to make it more reliable, for example using phone apps to get the timing as precise as possible.

The variety of methods available to meet different needs and preferences is astonishing, and the result of a huge research and development effort by public, private and voluntary organisations, with stringent controls from regulatory bodies to ensure safety as well as effectiveness. This is not to say that the list is perfect. Although the hormonal methods now use very small quantities compared with the early days of the contraceptive pill, many people would still prefer to avoid their use altogether and work is proceeding to develop a non-hormonal pill. There is also a need for a male contraceptive pill, which is quite difficult to achieve, and there is a new method, now undergoing trials, which uses a switch just under the skin of the scrotum to block or allow the flow of sperm into the ejaculate.

Although the range of possible methods is not perfect, in practice the contraceptive choices available are enough for most women and men to be able to avoid unwanted pregnancy safely and securely. In case of contraceptive failure, there is early termination of pregnancy through medical abortion (using mifepristone and mifepristone tablets) or a minor surgical abortion through vacuum aspiration, or dilatation and evacuation, as a day patient. In cases of foetal abnormality or a risk to the woman's life, a more serious surgical abortion may be used at a later stage. In most of the richer countries, these are available to those who want to avoid or terminate a pregnancy. In many poorer countries, they remain all too often a forbidden fruit and the only alternative is some kind of semi-poisonous medication or a crude surgical procedure, often without sterilisation of the instruments or pain relief for the woman. In some countries all abortion has been made illegal, or allowed only in the most traumatic cases of rape or a threat to the woman's life. Such moves do not stop women seeking abortions, they merely make it much more dangerous to do so.

Poor countries, good practice

Let us review three of the many hundreds of projects on different continents that are finding ways to bring modern methods to those who most need them, and then offer a few snapshots of innovative practice around the world. Any attempt to sum up the work being done is probably inadequate, given the scale and scope of it, but these offer a flavour of family planning in developing countries today.

Marie Stopes International (MSI) works in Tanzania, among many other countries, and has 11 clinics throughout the country's urban and peri-urban areas, serving a range of clients on middle to low incomes. With support from the Government of Tanzania, they are working to reduce the 7,900 deaths of women every year from pregnancy and childbirth, and the estimated one quarter of all women who have an unmet need for family planning.

In urban areas they use bajaji (a type of three-wheeled motorised rickshaw) to bring services at home to women who cannot get to the clinics. However many rural women in Tanzania are in even greater need, living in remote areas where clinics and hospitals are scarce, too expensive to reach, and often lacking appropriately trained staff and equipment. At these government-run facilities condoms and contraceptive pills may sometimes be available, but stocks frequently run out. Longer-acting (LARC) methods may be unaffordable, or rarely offered because staff do not know how to fit IUDs or implants, and may not have supplies.

A typical MSI rural team, in Kahama, includes one physician, two nurses, a driver and a government nurse, and uses specially equipped 4X4 vehicles to reach remote areas, holding sessions in local buildings or a blow-up marquee. Radio broadcasts and text messages tell people what is happening, and great care is taken to work with religious and other local leaders who can reassure their people that this is acceptable. Once assembled, the people are offered entertainment as well as information, through drama, comedy and group discussions. Often they use anatomical models, or pull out different types of contraception from their blue Choice Kits and demonstrate how to use them. People are encouraged to touch and hold these devices while hearing about what they do.

There have been many prejudices and misunderstandings about contraception in the outreach areas, with many believing it is bad for your health, or even makes you permanently infertile. The team may not change such opinions through a single session, but by returning many times with consistent, high-quality treatments that are obviously safe and effective, they can make contraception a real possibility for all. Women can also choose the method that will suit them best, with many going for the LARC methods. In cases where the men are opposed to contraception the women often choose injections, a method which is especially useful if they want to keep their treatment confidential from husbands and other family members who might try to stop it.

This kind of outreach is clearly working well. There are 600,000 clients for the family planning services and a reduced reliance on other unreliable methods such as condoms, as people switch to the more effective long-acting, reversible methods. This has prevented an estimated 920,000 unintended pregnancies and the death of 2,300 women. In addition, over 400 government health staff have been given training in modern family planning methods. However, a programme such as this is expensive to deliver. Until there are serious increases in funding for family planning it will not be available to all who need it. In the target areas there will perhaps be less need for educational work, as family planning and basic health care become more routine. Some resources can then be moved to other areas. However, this will take long-term and consistent funding and commitment, and the big question is whether international sources of aid will be able to sustain it.

In Guatemala the emphasis has been on working with traditional birth attendants, many of whom have inherited the role from other women in their own families, to work with the Mayan women of Santiago de Atitlan. Many of these Comadronas are older women who have worked for long periods in the region but received little training in modern methods. A small twice-weekly Comadrona School of POWHER (Providing Outreach for Women's Health Education and Resources) has been set up where techniques can be learned but, just as important, the women can discuss their own experiences and how to combine old traditions with modern methods.

A reporter from the US, herself medically qualified, was full of admiration for the women: "I was immediately humbled by the real world experience and skills these comadronas possess. They think through medical cases in the classroom, but their work takes place in the wider community." Invited to make home visits with them for ante-natal care, "While I found myself hesitant with my hands… the comadronas beside me channelled the knowledge they had gained from belonging to a cultural tradition and especially the school. They went about their work with confidence and care."

In Afghanistan, a different approach has been taken with a course set up for young people to study midwifery, including family planning. They all come from one of the most remote and hard-to-reach areas of Afghanistan, Daikundi, a mountainous region dotted with isolated green valleys. All of them have been selected by their neighbours, communities and village leaders to take a written exam, and the most successful are brought to Kabul for the course. The students and their families sign a commitment that they will return to the village once they finish their studies. Many of the young women come from families where their own mothers and grandmothers died in childbirth. One girl described the death of a woman in her community: "She lost a lot of blood and the placenta was retained. There was no midwife and she died. Her two children survived, but they died months later because the adopting families didn't have enough resources to take care of them."

The project, managed by the UN Fund for Population (UNFPA) in conjunction with the Afghan government and international aid donors, was set up after the people in local communities refused to accept mobile health teams and doctors. The new approach, according to Dr Molakhial of UNFPA, was intended to "actively involve the community in the process, guaranteeing their ownership from the very beginning". The project is a success because midwives return to their own communities with new skills, and also a new status. Each midwife runs a Family Health House that provides maternal, newborn and child health care for between 1,500 and 4,000 people.

The midwives also do outreach work with the community and with family decision-makers, to reach other girls and young women in their communities who are not getting access to information or health care. They are supported by mobile health teams offering technical and managerial assistance to the new midwives once or twice a month, and also providing vaccinations and other primary health care. There are 82 Family Health Houses and nine mobile health teams in three provinces, with nine more now coming into service.

These projects are just three examples out of hundreds of health and family planning programmes around the world: a mixture of high-quality medical interventions which can offer the best choice of methods with medical backup if needed, and locally based advocates and midwives who come from the community, know how to communicate with the people, and have their confidence. Whether it is Ita Ouali ("best friends") in the war-torn Central African Republic, midwives in displaced people's camps in Myanmar, or Lady Health Workers in Pakistan, recruiting and training local women is often the key to a successful programme. This can be especially important in areas of conflict, high migration, or refugee situations. The women and children involved are among the most vulnerable to abuse, exploitation and every kind of disadvantage.

Innovations

A number of initiatives have been developed by the UN Population Fund (UNFPA) for vulnerable young people, such as one in Mongolia. The "Y-Peer" scheme trains young volunteers to offer support to others who may be isolated, vulnerable and separated from their families in a rapidly changing society. They also offer information and access to health facilities, including contraception. One of the young teenagers they helped, who had been contemplating suicide, said, "Y-Peer saved my life. For that, I am so thankful."

In Nepal there is a programme in a remote region, Baitadi, where astrologers, shamans and priests have come together to persuade families not to force their children into premature marriage, sex and childbirth. When parents bring a girl's "cheena", an astrological chart, this is likely to mean preparations for her marriage. Astrologers say the parents often lie about their daughter's age, but the birth date on the cheena is always accurate. They can then advise the parents to delay the marriage until she reaches the legal marriage age of 20.

Also very important is relating to men in the community. Men typically want more children than women do, since they are not the ones bearing the personal and health costs of pregnancy and birth, and most play a lesser role in feeding and nurturing the children. Their understanding of the issues, however, can be crucial and there are many family planning programmes that reach out to the men for their support and participation. One example of this is the Schools for Husbands in rural Niger, West Africa, where modern contraception is only just starting to be introduced in many areas, and death rates for women are still extremely high. The country was ranked last on measures of gender equality in the 2013 Human Development Report, while men have been expected to take all the decisions in the household.

Starting in 2008, men have been invited to the local health centre to discuss issues of women's health and childbearing. When the initiative was launched, few thought it would succeed. "Years ago, it would have been difficult to talk about such issues with men in this village," said Almoustapha Boubacar, the manager of

Maiki health centre. Not all the men are invited: members must be married, at least 25, and accepting of women's participation in community life. These men become opinion-formers and role models within their communities, and some also work in collaboration with a group of women. They have provided some practical support to the health centres, and become effective in raising awareness in their communities about women's need for family planning and medical care for childbirth, although there are still some men who refuse even to discuss these issues. Meanwhile, the numbers of women coming to health centres has considerably increased in the areas where these schools for husbands are operating. Change can take a long time, but with help from a core of supportive men it is on the way.

Another innovative approach was the distribution of vouchers for women's health and contraceptive care. A scheme in Western Uganda sold vouchers at well below cost, redeemable against an approved list of high-quality services and medications for safe childbirth, treatment of infections and family planning. A previous trial had shown that using vouchers simplified the targeting of sales to the poor, minimised administration and controlled costs for the project overall. Voucher Community-Based Distributors (VCBDs) travelled around the villages to explain the benefits of using a clinic for delivery or to access other treatments. Using their local knowledge and the oral tradition of the villages they visited, VCBDs raised awareness of the scheme and generated lively community participation, with strong sales of the discounted vouchers. A problem arose when many of them left for a while to work for a political party in national elections. Overall, however, it was a great success.

The project set out to provide 50,456 safe deliveries and 35,000 treatments for sexually transmitted diseases (STDs). By

December 2011, when the project closed, more than 136,000 people had been independently verified as having received a range of reproductive health services. Mobile phone technology made project communications and data management more efficient and the project successfully demonstrated that critical project transactions can be sped up, and errors reduced, by using text messaging. A 2010 user satisfaction survey conducted by the Population Council found that 94% of voucher users said they were satisfied with the quality of health care services, compared with 76% of patients who did not use vouchers. The project's success resulted in the Government of Uganda committing additional funds of US$3 million to support the development of new voucher projects.

Another innovative project with potential for wider use is in Indonesia, where there was a family planning service but with relatively low quality. Yayasan Cipta Cara Padu works to involve leaders and statutory authorities at local level to implement the government's Kampung KB programme to revitalize and improve the existing programmes, with a particular emphasis on improving the range of choice of contraceptive methods and the quality of delivery and medical back-up.

Alongside these health promotion schemes, there are increasing numbers of smaller-scale Population, Health and Environment (PHE) projects, which use an integrated approach to preserve fragile environments and livelihoods. These use technical expertise and innovation for sustainable agriculture or fisheries through conservation of soil, water and wildlife, introducing alternative sources of income and improving hygiene and public health. Alongside this there are health services, including family planning, to help people to reduce unintended pregnancies and so relieve the pressure of increasing human numbers on those areas – in other words, to make them more sustainable for present and future generations.

One of the pioneers is Blue Ventures, in Madagascar. They are working on marine research and conservation: "We work in places where the ocean is vital to local cultures and economies, and are committed to protecting marine biodiversity in ways that benefit coastal people." They started by surveying coral reefs, where the local people were worried about the decline in their catches, and agreed with them to close off a small section of their octopus fishing area for a few months. When this was reopened there was a huge increase in landings and therefore people's incomes. As news spread, neighbouring communities started copying this approach and combined to create a locally managed Marine Area. Temporary fishery closures have now "gone viral" along much of the coastline of Madagascar. Alongside this there is a community health programme, known locally as Safidy or "Freedom to Choose". Local women are trained to offer family planning and other health services, selling contraceptives at a small profit, which they can keep for their own use. The health promoters are also offering basic health prevention measures such as mosquito nets, water purification equipment and oral rehydration salts for diarrhoea. The Blue Ventures outreach team regularly tours 32 coastal communities to discuss sexual and reproductive health, water purification and natural resource management. Smartphones are being introduced for communication and monitoring of the programme.

Telecommunications are also key to work in Nepal to provide support and counselling on sexual health matters through a free helpline called Meri Saathi ("My Friend"), advising on a wide range of issues from safe abortion, contraception and safe sex to masturbation, penis size and menstruation. In mountainous

Nepal, where it can take a woman days to get to the nearest primary health care centre, there is little accurate information. Sex before marriage is taboo, and so is discussion of sexual matters. The call centre is a lifeline for thousands of younger Nepalis. This is critical because, for example, abortion is legal during the first twelve weeks of pregnancy but many of the people do not know this. Dangerous abortion is still common and often self-inflicted with the insertion of iron bars, and the like, accounting for more than 5% of recorded maternal deaths.

The telephone service has proved very popular, going from 150 calls per month to 150 every day, and is being expanded. Many of the calls are from adolescent boys asking about masturbation as well as sex in general, while young women are mainly concerned about unwanted sexual advances and harassment, contraception, menstrual pain and access to safe abortions. Some are desperate to keep their contraceptive use secret from their husbands, who may be interested mainly in having sons, regardless of their wives' health and welfare. The success stories include a call centre operator persuading a mother not to force her 14-year-old daughter into marriage, and enabling thousands of women to avoid pregnancy when the time is not right for them to have a child.

Publicity

Communications – this time in the form of soap operas – lie behind some of the most interesting initiatives in this field. Even where people have access to family planning, social attitudes and prejudices may mean that there is a lack of confidence in it: fear of side effects, religious opposition and couples' inability to talk to each other about sex and pregnancy. To get people thinking realistically about these issues, TV and radio drama series have proved very effective. The Population Media Centre produces locally written dramas in which key characters embrace such things as family planning, schooling for girls and other social and health issues. Researchers typically spend weeks talking to people in the target community, identifying the issues that matter to them.

The idea of combining melodrama and public health was first developed in Mexico in the 1970s by Miguel Sabido, a television executive who believed that national welfare mattered as much as ratings. His shows promoting literacy and family planning became smash hits and generated impressive impacts. The year Sabido's first program, *Ven Conmigo*, appeared, the number of people signing up for government literacy classes jumped more than eight times. Following the run of a second show, *Acompáñame*, sales of over-the-counter contraception spiked by 23%. Radio and television dramas inspired by Sabido's model have now appeared in dozens of countries. "This is not a one-hour after-school special, or a one-minute public-service announcement," says Arvind Singhal, a professor of communication at the University of Texas-El Paso who has researched the impact of such shows. "These are programs that play themselves out over hundreds of episodes. If the programme is good, then you not only grab attention, but you grab it over a period of time."

There is evidence of dramatic results in the 45 countries in which the programmes have aired. For example, in northern Nigeria a radio serial was heard regularly by more than 70% of the population, and a study found that about two thirds of those seeking contraception cited the programme as a motivating factor. Those who listened to the programme also reported wanting fewer children than before. In Ethiopia, during the two and a half years a similar programme was broadcast, 40% of listeners reported using modern contraceptive methods compared with 25% of non-listeners. Communications of course have to be accompanied by good service provision, otherwise people can simply be frustrated when they want to try to make changes.

Sometimes even adverse publicity can work. A few years ago when the injectable contraceptive Depo Provera was first made available, there was a campaign against it in some European countries, some of it inspired by pro-lifers. They exaggerated the supposedly awful side effects and called for it to be banned, especially in developing countries. The attacks on Depo were repeatedly aired on radio and TV in Tanzania. Clinics there were amazed when women started queuing round the block for it. It seems the women got the message about preventing unwanted pregnancies and saw this as far outweighing any fears about side effects. Perhaps they were hearing the awful warnings about this new contraceptive in the way that the Kremlinologists of the Cold War used to read and listen to Soviet media: ignoring the propaganda while looking for clues to the real situation.

Governments

Many of the programmes outlined above are successful because they have the backing of the national governments, even though most of the funds, expertise and personnel are brought in from outside. Increasingly, governments of developing countries are starting to perceive the importance of modern contraception for their countries' future welfare and prosperity. From the very poorest (Bangladesh, Bhutan, Ethiopia) to the strongly Muslim (Iran, Indonesia, Malaysia) or Catholic (Mexico) and with the worst history of ethnic conflict (Rwanda) to middle-income countries (South Korea, Thailand), governments have shown that good family planning policies and programmes are possible. Among the most improved countries in this regard are two African states, Sierra Leone and Lesotho – both of which have emerged from a background of conflict and extreme poverty.

Where there is almost universal access to contraceptive services, the disadvantage suffered by the poorest women almost disappears and this is a serious contribution to increased equality among households. It is also a factor in economic growth. The Republic of Korea is an example of the "tiger economies" of Asia, which have managed to turn their countries around. "Investments in health, including reproductive health services, coupled with investments in education, contributed to an economic 'miracle', opening opportunities for all," according to the latest review by the UNFPA. It is often forgotten that Japan, too, achieved its "economic miracle" after the disasters of the Second World War and a post-war "baby boom" by promoting family planning and legalising abortion.

In Bangladesh, one of the poorest and most densely populated countries in the world, 61% of currently married women in a 2100 survey said that they were using some form of family planning, a level comparable to developed countries, and the total fertility rate has declined steadily to 2.3 children per woman.

One of the most striking success stories is that of a small Pacific island nation, the Maldives. We might think that being a small country, to improve women's and children's health and survival rates and offer modern family planning would be simple. In fact it is very difficult because of the problems of serving many small and scattered islands. The 25-year campaign to improve women's reproductive health, with a family planning campaign and huge improvements in obstetric care, has resulted in a remarkable 90% drop in maternal death rates. The Health Ministry initiated in-depth reviews of all maternal deaths, helping planners to understand the causes. Health workers then received additional training and were deployed within the islands and atolls to provide home visits. Close monitoring proved essential, particularly for women with high-risk pregnancies. At the same time family planning information and access were improved. Community health workers made home visits to tell women about the benefits of planning their pregnancies. The government disseminated information via the mass media, using dramas and songs about all aspects of reproductive health from contraception to nutrition and safe childbirth. UNFPA increased the quantity and variety of contraceptive products available, including male and female condoms, oral contraceptives, intra-uterine devices and implants. This is an outstanding example of local, national and international organisations working together over an extended period of time to turn around a disastrous situation for women and make this country one of the best for health in the developing world.

If they can do it, any country can. The tragedy is that for far too many, there is still nothing being done.

Considering coercion

There have in the past been so-called "family planning" programmes based not on choice but on coercion. They have demonstrated that they are not only wrong in principle, but also counter-productive, giving contraception a bad name in areas where incentives or penalties have been used. An obvious example is that of government programmes in India, which set up sterilisation camps and either offered people money to accept the operation or gave financial inducements to officials to gather people in without explaining what sterilisation was. Medical backup was clearly lacking, or very inadequate. The result was an enormous amount of distress among people who perhaps did not understand that this was a permanent end to their fertility but also had little or no choice about whether to accept it. Too many people suffered greatly from health complications. The programme sparked an angry resistance to the idea of all family planning in the areas concerned, and helped to make the notion of "population control" even more of a taboo subject internationally.

What is less recognised is that the programme operated mainly in north India, while in the south of the country programmes were voluntary and were well accepted by people. This, combined with the greater autonomy of many women in the south, contributed to the wide gulf in fertility rates that prevails between north and south India now, and the social and economic benefits now being felt in the south.

The other, and most important, case of enforced contraception is of course China, the country with the biggest population in the world. Its "one child" policy for many Chinese families was notorious for its cruelty. Women were forced to abort female foetuses, and newborn girls were often abandoned because the family insisted that the one child must be a boy. Sex selection has also led to a huge imbalance in the ratio of boys to girls, with all the social tensions caused by this. Unknown numbers of babies were born who became "non-persons", unable to become legal citizens and excluded from education and social support because their parents could not pay the fine or bribe for the "extra" child and therefore could not register the birth. Unmarried women and couples were also fined if they had a baby, and their child was also excluded from registration.

The Chinese policy has been accompanied by rampant corruption as implementation of this government policy was left to the provinces. Many local officials demanded bribes for allowing children to be born and registered, favouring some families while penalising those who resisted. The policy, which always had exemptions for ethnic minorities and rural areas, has now been modified to allow two children per couple. However, the official controls on people's choices about pregnancy and birth remain in place. It has been argued that all this was completely unnecessary since birth rates were already declining rapidly before the "one child" policy was introduced, and the same effort put into good health provision and family planning choices could have resulted in a similar drop in family size and therefore the national population.

The other example of government attempts to force people to limit the size of their families is Myanmar, which has tried to impose this on the Rohingya minority. This soon developed into a programme of forced evictions and the burning of villages, accompanied by horrific violence and the deliberate killing of large numbers of Rohingyas, targeting babies and children as well as adults, in a campaign that has been described as genocide.

Coercion has no place in family planning programmes: personal choice must be the key. The case of China and its notorious "one child" policy has served to discredit the cause of family planning internationally, and especially in the rest of Asia. Let's hope they move as quickly as possible to allowing the people, not the State, to plan their own families.

Conclusions: more work still needed
Perhaps one of the most crucial indicators of progress is the willingness of so many organisations and governments to learn

from experience and to evaluate what works best and how programmes can be improved. In a landmark report from the FP2020 (Family Planning 2020)) campaign run by UNFPA with money from the Gates Foundation, they reveal that some of the targets – 120 million additional users by 2020, with universal access to modern contraception by 2030 – are falling short at the half-way mark, and require some serious work on the bottlenecks if the final goals are to be achieved.

"The richness of the data now available enables us to peel back the layers and study the situation on a country-by-country basis. What emerges is a strikingly varied landscape of progress. A number of countries have registered immense gains in contraceptive use; other countries are moving more slowly; some countries appear stalled... This knowledge is part of the toolkit we take into the second half of the initiative. We also bring with us a deeper understanding of how family planning services reach, or fail to reach, specific sub-populations of women and girls. The evidence base is growing for a wide range of issues and interventions, including youth-oriented approaches, method mix diversity, stock-outs, contraceptive discontinuation, rights-based programming, and postpartum family planning. The resulting insights can help us shape more effective programs, investments, and policies to reach women and girls with the services they need." They also point to three other main areas for future focus: accountability in terms of returns on money invested and the assessment of outcomes; partnerships, making donors work more effectively with government and co-operating better with each other; and youth, meeting the urgent contraceptive needs of young people in new and more effective ways.

There is a dilemma here, and it is largely a financial one: we would all want the widest range of contraceptive choices, backed by state-of-the-art obstetric and gynaecological health facilities and medical backup. Enormous amounts of work have been done to make this possible and much more affordable for individual users. And yet the money is not there to achieve this in all parts of the world at the same time. US Government opposition to allowing aid programmes to fund family planning is also relentless, as we shall discuss in Part Two.

A bad atmosphere around this issue is also created by is the constant scrutiny of services by opponents to discover any shortfall in care, real or often imaginary, that they can broadcast to the world as evidence for their claim that family planning is itself harmful and wrong. The truth is that no medical procedures are perfect. Meanwhile, the horrific record of deaths and injuries where there are no such services is never mentioned by the opposition. The UNFPA points out that countries with low rates of family planning services for the poorest women also have the least adequate antenatal and maternity services, and very high death rates for women and babies.

It is critically important that we continue working to ensure the highest levels of effectiveness and safety within the very limited budgets that are being allocated to this. At the same time these budgets need to be greatly increased if real choice is to be achieved everywhere it is needed.

Lives depend on it. The work goes on.

Resources

"What are the different types of contraception?" United States Department of Health and Human Development, National Institutes of Health website.

For details of family planning programmes see the websites of UNFPA, Marie Stopes International, and, FP2020 (Advance Family Planning) and other aid providers. Family Planning 2020 (FP2020), part-funded by the Gates Foundation, is also doing important research and programme work.

Bangladesh 2011, *Demographic and Health Survey.*

UNFPA, *The State of World Population 2017.*

FP2020, *Momentum at the Midpoint 2015-2016.*

PART TWO:
THE ISSUES

Chapter three

"GET BREEDING…"
Modern eugenics: racism, nationalism, fundamentalism

Eugenics: it is meant to be a word to strike terror in the heart of those who advocate any kind of free choice when it comes to having babies. It is sometimes claimed that our promotion of contraception, leading to fewer births, is really promoting a policy of selective human breeding controls that are somehow in conformity with the racial policies of Nazi Germany. The reality is the exact opposite of this: the modern advocates of eugenics promote maximum births in their own particular group through opposition to choice through family planning. Eugenics always means coercion, depriving individuals of any ability to make their own decisions about their families. Voluntary, informed family planning – enabling control by women and their partners – is the opposite of eugenics.

The early "eugenic" ideas of the late 19th and early 20th centuries meant changing the population by promoting births among some people while stopping or discouraging births among others. There were certainly strong racist overtones to some of the debate, with some claiming that "Europeans" were superior to any others. Others thought humanity could be "improved" by eugenics. The idea was promoted by people of both the Right and the Left for very different reasons, ranging from helping individual women to controlling whole populations. They included such notables as the black rights advocate WEB DuBois and the economist John Maynard Keynes. Some advocates of family planning, notably Margaret Sanger in the US, used the language of eugenics to further the cause of individual choice, possibly as a defence against vicious attacks on early family planning advocates by right-wingers who opposed contraception on principle. Those people argued that "the races of northern Europe" were "doomed to extinction, unless each family produces at least four children," as one Catholic bishop and eugenicist wrote to her.

The Nazis picked up this extreme right wing and racist version of eugenics and made it their own. They went much further than the previous advocates, of course, killing millions of people they considered the wrong "race" while encouraging or even forcing women of their own nationality they called "Aryans" to bear the maximum number of children possible.

It is important to understand what the Nazis' eugenic policy really meant: this was at the heart of their theories and not some fringe idea, and it was played out in the lives and deaths of millions of people. Heimlich Himmler, using his elite SS troops, organised the systematic destruction of huge numbers of babies and children, starting with disabled or "defective" children in Germany itself. Once extended across Europe, their eugenic policies focused especially on Jewish and Roma people, especially children, but also many of the Slavic "race" in eastern Europe. They murdered them inside the concentration camps and in the killing fields outside, often alongside their mothers. Millions of people in the occupied countries were also starved, and excluded from any kind of medical treatment.

It was this same Himmler who organised the Lebensborn (Fountain of Life) programme intended to produce racially and ideologically "pure" children for the Nazi cause. Half a million children from all over Europe who were judged "racially correct" were taken away from their families and placed in the SS Lebensborn institutions, where they were treated very harshly in an attempt to indoctrinate them as Nazi soldiers. Many German babies were also taken from their families to be brought up there. The surviving children, now in their 60s and beyond, say they have felt "lost" for their whole lives, the result of being used as pawns in a racist eugenics ideology. Those taken to the institutions as toddlers talk of sitting on the windowsills endlessly looking out, hoping that their mother or father would come for them.

The racist attitude to babies and children was not confined to the elite but was deeply entrenched among Nazi soldiers. A new book on German prisoners of war, drawing on their secretly recorded conversations, reveals that the majority saw Roma (Gypsies), Jews, gays and the disabled as "useless mouths" that deserved to die. They expressed particular hatred of the women and children, whom they feared and hated even more than the enemy soldiers.

Nazi policies on contraception and abortion have been researched by the feminist leader Gloria Steinem. She found them strongly opposed to any choice for German women:

"Hitler himself, and the Nazi doctrine he created, were unequivocally opposed to any individual right to abortion. In fact Hitler's National Socialist Movement preached against and punished contraception, homosexuality, women whose main purpose was not motherhood, men who did not prove their manhood by fathering many children – and anything else that failed to serve the need of preserving and expanding the German state. There were tax penalties for being unmarried, payments for childbearing, and the prohibition of contraception and abortion, as well as homosexuality. Those performing terminations faced a possible death penalty. In 1933 feminists were removed from teaching and other public posts by the same law that removed 'non-Aryans' from such jobs." She quotes Adolf Hitler himself as the prime advocate of eugenics in Germany: "Every child that a woman brings into the world is a battle, a battle waged for the existence of her people..."

It is ironic that advocates of contraception are often accused by the opposition of being eugenicists. In fact it is the pro-natalists, who want to persuade or force women to bear children, who are preaching eugenics in a modern context, and often seeking to ban all forms of family planning. Put simply, they are arguing for increases in their own group's population in competition with other groups, perhaps killing the others or forcing them out of their homes and lands. They are prepared to use their own children as cannon fodder in sectarian conflicts. In a war situation they kill children of the "other" side, or abduct those children and force them to fight, and in extreme cases even to commit atrocities against their own people in order to stay alive themselves. For terrorist groups using suicide bombings there have been reports of children being used to carry explosives, often without any understanding of the horror they are getting into. For such people it is only the numbers of children that counts – individuals are expendable. Forced childbirth for women in their own group is the flipside of genocide against others, just as the Nazis before them.

There is tragic evidence from other conflicts that babies and children are seen as particular targets by some regimes and militia groups. In Syria, for example, there have been reports of government aircraft deliberately bombing groups of children playing outside. In Myanmar, government troops are reported to have thrown babies onto fires or smashed their heads on the ground before attacking the women. In the Central African Republic, the Seleka militia groups have killed large numbers of women with children. A first-aid worker reported in 2013 that in the village of Bombi Te armed militia first robbed his wife, then ordered her to leave while they attacked her four-year-old child. "They tried to shoot him but the gun was not working. So they slit his throat instead. What threat does this child pose to the Seleka? He is just a child."

"The punishment is motherhood"

Advocates of forcing women to bear more children are getting louder, and Europe and the US – where most women now have access to a range of contraception – seem to be hotspots for this. Jonathan V Last, the US author of *What to Expect When No One's Expecting,* claims that his people are having "too few babies". He argues: "If America wants to continue to lead the world, we need to have more babies." Conservative British commentator Charles Moore says: "You can borrow and spend hugely if you know that the generation that will end up with the bill is much larger than your own. If it is much smaller, you can't; but we have. As a result, Europe is a dying business. Most of the world is not. So it is winning… Meanwhile, get breeding."

There has been a flurry of other overtly racist books published in the United States, some of them bestsellers, which claim that because the population of Europe in particular is not increasing, or not fast enough, they face catastrophe. They claim that people of other religions and "races" will increase their numbers more rapidly and somehow overwhelm the native population. Pat Buchanan, in *The Death of the West*, claims that "the rise of feminism spells the death of the nation and the end of the West." Mark Steyn in *America Alone* predicts "the demise of European races too self-absorbed to breed. In demographic terms, the salient feature of much of the 'progressive agenda' – abortion, gay marriage, endlessly deferred adulthood [means]… as fertility dries up, so do societies." This word "breeding" is one used for domestic animals produced for human consumption and use, and is wholly inappropriate for our fellow humans.

The numbers they most want to increase are fellow conservatives. Here is David Bentley Hart, a conservative Catholic theologian in the US: "Probably the most subversive and effective strategy we might undertake would be one of militant fecundity: abundant, relentless, exuberant, and defiant childbearing. Given the reluctance of modern men and women to be fruitful and multiply, it would not be difficult, surely, for the devout to accomplish – in no more than a generation or two – a demographic revolution."

He is referring to the Catholic Church's expansion in opposition to Protestants, members of other faiths, and non-believers. Perhaps more precisely, since most Catholics now use contraception and have small families, it is a call to use women to grow the militant conservative faction within the church at the expense of the liberals. Membership is seen as a battle of the numbers. Once a Catholic community is established, especially in the developed countries, conversion to the faith is uncommon so church membership will grow almost entirely through the numbers of babies its members have. This must be an important factor in the hierarchy's insistence on opposing birth planning or choice, and giving this priority over purely moral issues.

The "get breeding" order might all seem a bit of a joke – a few ultra-conservatives ranting and raving while most people simply ignore what they have to say and make their own decisions. But in many parts of the world it is deadly serious. Many ethnic, cultural and religious rivalries, many of them spilling over into war, are stoked by the perception that "they" are breeding and "we" are not, or at least not fast enough. Since this is very largely a male argument (and since they have not yet worked out how to make babies on their own) it means heavy pressure on girls and women to marry early and face a lifetime of pregnancies and childbirth, while contraception is made unavailable and terminations are made highly dangerous.

Some revolutionaries and left-wingers are also quite similar in their views on this to the conservatives, though for their own reasons: having more children to fight in their wars or vote for them in elections. Michelle Goldberg describes how Daniel Ortega, formerly the leader of the Sandinistas in Nicaragua, went on to win an election based partly on his support for continuing a ban on abortion brought in by his conservative predecessors. When a group of Sandinista women and men presented him with a declaration on sexual rights, including access to contraception, abortion and sex education, he told them to forget it "because we have to replace the fifty thousand martyrs of the revolution".

Islamist and other terror groups are also keen to get as many children for their own group as possible, while not hesitating to kill the babies and children of others. Indeed Da'esh (Isis) has invested much energy in recruiting girls and young women from western countries to come and marry their fighters and produce babies for the cause. They have also used captured women of Yazidi, Christian and other groups, who are raped and then forced to bear the children that result.

Conflict

Many of the countries with repressive laws against contraception and abortion have a background of ethnic or religious tensions and conflicts. Northern Ireland, for example, with its extreme sensitivities over population numbers of Catholics and Protestants, has an almost total legal ban on abortion, and a culture of enforced motherhood, coming from people on both sides of the religious divide. This is in spite of it being part of the United Kingdom, which otherwise has liberal policies on abortion.

One pro-choice campaigner in Northern Ireland described the attitudes of many to pregnant women: "There just seems to be this huge culture of shame. This idea that oh, you had sex, you are a dirty slut, the punishment is motherhood." As the Peruvian pro-choice activist Kelly Cieza puts it: "Motherhood cannot be imposed as an obligation or punishment." Sadly, in too many areas it can be, and it is. How can they use childbirth and the care of a baby as punishment? The consequences for women and children are incalculable.

The battles are still raging even in many of the richer countries with mainly liberal law and social policy, but the situation is worse – much worse – for women facing the new eugenics being imposed in many developing countries. In Nigeria, for example, the question of how many people there are, in which region of the country or in which ethnic or religious group, is too sensitive for even a proper census. Politicians of different groups have exploited the fear that "the others" are greater in number, will get more resources, and are increasing faster. The result: very few options for women to plan the birth of their children, high rates of enforced pregnancy and childbirth, and extremely high mortality rates. Overall population numbers have tripled since independence in 1960, and could double again in less than 25 years. As a result of its ethnic conflicts, Nigeria has one of the highest rates of pregnancy and childbirth in the world.

Intense pressure on women to bear more children is a particular feature of colonial and settler movements. In the colonisation period in what is now the United States, for example, birth rates were exceptionally high – far exceeding those in Europe, from which the settlers had recently arrived. At the same time, the numbers of Native Americans were drastically cut by massacres and wars, disease, environmental destruction and the theft of their lands and livelihoods. Their numbers east of the Mississippi River fell from an estimated two million in 1492 to just a quarter of a million in 1750 – that is, three quarters of the population died. The same or similar phenomenon can be found in many expansionist societies today which are seeking to drive out the inhabitants of other groups, whether through violence or by the sheer weight of their own group's numbers.

Fundamentalism

The concept of "fundamentalism" was coined as a term for Christian evangelicals in the United States in the early 20th century who were fighting for the "fundamentals of faith" in the face of modern ideas. It can now be applied to a particular use (or rather abuse) of religion across the whole spectrum. Women's organisations have identified fundamentalist groups in Catholic and other Christian churches, Buddhist, Hindu, Jewish and Sikh religions, as well as local ethno-religious traditions such as the Kenyan Mungiki movement, Mexican indigenous Tepehuan, Nepali shamanism, and new religions or cults such as the Moonies' Unification Church which has arranged marriages for thousands of its younger members.

A fairly typical example of the sectarian attitudes of these groups is from MS Golwalkar, an architect of the "Hindutva" (Hinduness) ideology: "The non-Hindu people of Hindustan must either adopt Hindu culture and language, must learn and respect and hold in reverence the Hindu religion, must entertain no idea but of those of glorification of the Hindu race and culture or may stay in the country wholly subordinated to the Hindu nation, deserving no privileges, far less any preferential treatment – not even citizens' rights." A common theme here, and of fundamentalists in general, is a hatred and scorn for the idea of universal human rights, and particularly women's rights.

With the exception of some cults, the fundamentalists do not represent their whole religion. They operate a distortion of their faith, their own version of which they claim to be "the Truth". While fundamentalists appear to disagree violently with each other and are in conflict on many issues, a common theme among them is controlling "their" women, and especially pregnancies and childbearing, in order to maximise the number of "their" children. A militantly male phenomenon (although women can be co-opted), it represents both a reactionary backlash against the women's movement and a distancing or even contempt, among the men involved, for all women, our bodies, feelings and wishes.

The Anglican commentator Reverend Giles Fraser, who often has to deal with Christian Protestant fundamentalists, describes them as "locked in a self-referencing worldview where truth is about strict internal coherence rather than any reaching out to reality," selectively using texts from the Bible to fit their theories. It might more appropriately be seen as an extreme authoritarianism. Their logic is: "I have authority over everyone else, especially the women, because I can claim these sacred texts and ancient traditions. These are absolute and not open to question or discussion. Therefore my orders cannot be questioned..." It is an individual pathology, which is translated into a demand for implacable loyalty to the group and to themselves personally.

As one feminist from Argentina has put it, "Speaking with the support of God is something very different from speaking without it... It puts [women] on the side of sin and the Devil." Nira Yuval-Davis, an observer of the phenomenon in conservative Judaism, calls it "a political use of religion". "This version of religion, because it tends to be pre-modern and talk about 'purification' and going back to the 'Truth', latches on to patriarchal modes of society and control of women." She adds that some women in the Israeli settler movement take it on themselves as a patriotic or religious duty to have as many children as possible. "The role of the mother is absolutely central, in a kind of sacrificial role for the settlement" although the movement is controlled by the men. Meanwhile, the late Palestinian leader Yasser Arafat described his biggest weapon as "the womb of the Arab woman". In the context of the Arab-Israeli conflict all this would be farcical if it were not so tragic in terms of human lives and any prospect of peace.

A Muslim cleric in Iran, Mojtaba Takhtipour, interviewed by the *New York Times*, said that Islam orders a quest for a perfect society. "That means we need to increase the number of Muslims, so we also need more kids." To those who worry about supporting large numbers of children, he argues: "We do believe that ultimately God will provide our daily bread. So go out and have kids and have faith, is what I always say." This is far from the accepted view throughout Islam, but since there is no central religious authority there can be many different authorities and interpretations.

Feminist observers of fundamentalism see it not as some genuine survival from pre-modern times but as a very modern reaction to events in the world today, and especially the fight for resources. Most fundamentalists, they argue, are not really retreating into the past: they use modern technologies to spread their message including the internet, cable TV and satellite communications. They also operate trans-nationally, using modern media, perhaps to bypass opposition they may face at home. The Association for Women's Rights in Development (AWID) has surveyed 1,600 women's rights activists facing fundamentalist opposition. They conclude that the fundamentalists are extremely right wing politically, absolutist and intolerant, with a "conviction that they are divinely mandated to impose on others what they believe to be the singular truth".

Not all fundamentalist groups are violent, but those that are do not hesitate to attack other people, either verbally and sometimes with the threat or use of force. The main targets are likely to be members of other groups and other religions, or none, while people within their own community may also be subject to pressure if they refuse to accept their ideas. Extreme fundamentalists will often attack their own co-religionists precisely because they have little real depth of support within their own community. A human rights activist from Egypt told AWID researchers: "In most cases when people are offered an alternative interpretation, they take it, because they say it's a suffocating life to live as is preached by those religious fundamentalists." The position of the Catholic hierarchy also comes to mind, where they have failed to convince their own members on "Life" issues but devote great efforts to persuading politicians nationally and internationally to block women's rights, for Catholics and non-Catholics alike, and especially on fertility issues.

The AWID study concludes that among fundamentalists, "women are conceptualized as the reproducers and symbols of a community's collective identity" and therefore of its influence and power. "This translates into an obsession with the control of women's bodies and autonomy" with particular emphasis on restricting choice about having children, imposing a strict "morality" on women, and imposing a rigid definition of women's and men's roles in the family and society. Many of them are particularly hostile to sexual non-conformists such as lesbians, gay men and transsexuals. In Mongolia for example there are increasing threats coming from ultra-nationalist groups and religious fundamentalists to stop abortion, which is currently legal, claiming that women should produce more babies to ensure national security and sustain the so-called "pure Mongolian blood." In Thailand, it is militant Buddhist fundamentalists taking a similar line. The pattern is repeated in many other countries across the world.

Most fundamentalists are actively recruiting, especially among young and disaffected people who are looking for a cause and an identity, and many of them specialise in offering education and membership of their youth organisations. Their absolutist message can be very appealing to young people, especially boys and men who are seeking a strong identity for themselves, some power over women, and a role and purpose in society; they can then be mobilised for the cause. In this way AWID describes fundamentalists, where they are strong, as "effectively influencing society without having to capture state power".

Is this war?

The fundamentalists of all major religions are of course competing with each other to recruit more and more members, especially in areas with sectarian tensions. With both sides trying to increase their numbers by persuading or forcing the women to have big families, there can be a kind of arms race of childbirth. In the Middle East generally, there is increasing conflict between Sunnis, the majority who also have the highest birth rate, and Shias who generally have much smaller families. Da'esh (ISIS), which is Sunni-based, have put great efforts into using the internet to groom and recruit Muslim women from other countries to travel to occupied areas to marry their fighters and produce as many babies as possible. They have also kidnapped enormous numbers of Yazidi and other women from areas they have occupied, and subjected them to systematic rape, sale as sex slaves, and forcing them to bear children for their controllers.

Competition for numbers has been suggested as the main reason for the Catholic hierarchy's emphasis on political authority over so-called "Life" issues. For centuries they have had a vigorous missionary effort to set up new churches in areas of the developing world. Since the Reformation in Europe and the creation of Protestant churches they have had an intense rivalry over the number of their members. They now face intense competition with rapidly growing evangelical churches, especially in Latin America, where Catholics are defecting to them in large numbers. Some of these evangelicals – especially some of the conservative US-based ones – are themselves fundamentalists who promote conventional roles for women, which would of course include producing many children and bringing them up within the church.

At the same time, religious fundamentalists are also competing with secular movements such as left wing political parties or other opposition groups. In the many totalitarian countries that cannot tolerate organised opposition, political parties have been savagely repressed and this has left the field clear for the religious organisations. In many cases fundamentalist groups survive and thrive in poor areas by offering basic medical or welfare services – but no family planning. The condition of any help, of course, is loyalty to them and at least tacit acceptance of their doctrines.

Fundamentalists have always been with us, if only as a personality type which says "I know best, and how dare you question me?" What is new in the modern world is the political clout they have accumulated, especially as they use modern mass media and ally themselves with conservative and nationalist forces generally. Many of them are well funded, and may have great influence over governments. Fundamentalist Christians and the "Tea Party" movement in the US have scored a major victory with the election of Donald Trump as President. Variations on this theme can be found, among many others, with Catholic hierarchies in the Philippines and much of Latin America, Buddhist fundamentalists in Myanmar (Burma), Da'esh (ISIS), al-Qa'eda and allied "Islamist" groups controlling whole areas in the Middle East, Somalia and parts of West Africa, or Hindu fundamentalists attacking Muslims in India or Muslims attacking religious minorities in Pakistan.

In extreme cases sectarian fundamentalists will use extreme violence, up to and including murder, to silence criticism especially from human rights workers. Several women defenders of human rights have been killed or badly injured by fundamentalists. Nearly 10% of women's rights activists have experienced attacks on their offices or theft of their equipment, according to the AWID survey.

This violence has sometimes been turned on non-political humanitarian organisations, especially health workers who help women. Vaccination campaigns against polio have been a particular target. In northern Nigeria, for example, at least nine women were shot dead while working on a programme to immunise children against polio, and several doctors were also murdered. This was blamed on the Islamist militia group Boko Haram. The campaign against immunisation is linked to claims by some Imams that the drops are contaminated, as part of a "western campaign" to sterilise young girls and wipe out the whole Muslim population. The result of this and other attacks and scares was an epidemic of polio which has led to hundreds of children being infected, with many dying and others being so severely disabled that they can only survive by begging in the streets. This is at a time when the disease had been eliminated from almost every other country in the world. India, for example, has achieved a complete eradication of polio after an exhaustive campaign.

Polio eradication campaigns and health services are also targets for Islamists in the Peshawar area of Pakistan. Eight health workers were killed there in a single week in 2013, including those taking part in an ambitious drive to immunise millions of children against polio. This followed claims by the Taliban that the anti-polio work was part of a western plot to sterilise women.

At the heart of the conflict in Pakistan are Lady Health Workers (LHWs), a force of 110,000 women set up by the late Benazir Bhutto when she was Prime Minister, to help women and children. They are specifically tasked with visiting women at home to provide general health and contraceptive services, since many are not allowed to visit clinics on their own. These health workers have become a prime target for Taliban and other Islamist groups in Pakistan, with threats of kidnapping, rape and in some cases death. The most intimidating tactic is to "name and shame" individual women working in health, using radio broadcasts to issue *fatwas* against them personally. These declared that "it is a Muslim man's duty" to kidnap the women health workers when they paid home visits, to force them into marriages even if they were already married women, or to use them as sexual slaves. In the Swat region, which the Taliban occupied for three years up to 2009, their chief Maulana Fazlullah even declared LHWs to be "fit for murder". Some were indeed executed, publicly beaten, or their family members were murdered.

The threats against LHWs in Swat understandably forced many of them to resign, stop working or flee the area, and their patients suffered badly as a result. A study by the *British Medical Journal* found an increased number of deaths in childbirth, forced marriages and dangerous abortions. They quote one supervisor: "A lot of people stopped using family planning methods. They said it's against Islam. They got pregnant. Now the Taliban are gone they are aborting the pregnancies. Abortions are on the rise and women are dying."

Horrifying as this is, it is important to note that Islamist paranoia about health workers has been increased by incidents where western military units, including special forces, have hidden behind health and other aid projects. This has increased suspicion of all aid projects and made it much more dangerous for them to do their work. US special forces set up a "dummy" polio immunisation scheme as cover for their tracking and murder of al-Qa'eda chief Osama bin Laden. The damage done by this to health programmes, especially for women, is enormous and the tactic cannot be justified. It is essential that all military forces stop using health and aid programmes as cover for their own activities. It will take a long time for trust to be fully restored.

Pakistan had previously been a pioneer of family planning, the second country (after India) ever to initiate a national programme. Fundamentalists have now managed to entrench the idea, especially in rural areas, that using contraception is "un-Islamic", and as a result the country is now one of the least successful in offering services. "Family planning is a Western ideology to stop women from giving birth completely," one Islamist told BBC News. Almost all the women in Pakistan who use modern contraception are urban and educated, while those most in need of the services have little or no access.

This is in stark contrast to the fact that some of the most successful countries in this field – notably Iran, Bangladesh and Indonesia – are Muslim-majority states, and all have strong Islamic government identities. One important factor is that they have religious parties that have more enlightened attitudes, for example the Jamaat in Bangladesh which has no policy of opposing choice. They are among those who accept the original teachings of Islam: there is consensus among scholars that neither Quranic verses nor the Hadith contain any instructions on contraception. In fact Muslim governments have historically allowed contraception and abortion, for example in the Ottoman Empire and in Egypt. As with historical Catholic thought, it was believed that the foetus did not undergo "ensoulment" to become a human being until 120 days after conception.

In Pakistan, what appears to be a religious issue may be better described as political, with a struggle for influence between different groups. Two major Islamic political parties, JUI-F and Jamaat-e-Islami, have opposed choice since the 1930s. As Dr

Mehtab Karim has pointed out, the "vote bank" for the hard-line Islamic parties will increase from about 85 million people in 2013 to over 105 million in the next five years because of their pro-natalist policies. Almost all of these people will be very poor and illiterate – perfect voting fodder to maintain and increase hard-line political influence.

Similar calculations seem to underlie the position of other Islamist parties and some Islamist governments, where political power rests on the number of supporters. For example the Muslim Brotherhood, when in power in Egypt, denounced the proposed "Agreed Conclusions" of the UN Commission on the Status of Women, which called for sexual and reproductive rights for women, as "the intellectual and cultural invasion of Muslim countries" that would undermine Islamic ethics and "destroy the family".

Many women's groups, clerics and scholars in Islamic countries are contesting such fundamentalist dictates, often at considerable personal risk. During the Arab Spring uprising and subsequent protests in Egypt women played a key role, coming out in huge numbers to demonstrate for a democratic future. They were targeted by organised gangs of men who picked out women for sexual assault and rape, often leading to severe injuries. These men were identified as Muslim Brotherhood members and Salafists operating in a systematic, pre-planned way: around 15–20 men would surround one or two women, then up to 50 men would join in. The inner group would strip, molest and rape the women, and the outer group would fight anyone trying to rescue them. Under Morsi's Muslim Brotherhood government, no action was taken to prevent these assaults and no arrests or prosecutions undertaken, even where the perpetrators were identified. Indeed, there were incidents where the security forces helped the Islamists hold on to their "captured women". Was this a war against women? Apparently, for the Islamists, it was.

Women activists around the world are bravely confronting fundamentalists of all stripes. One of many examples is Musarrat Shaheen, a tribal woman and former film star from the DI Khan area near the Afghan border, which is plagued by extremist violence. Standing for election to the national parliament in Pakistan, she is contemptuous of the male religious leaders – a feeling that stems from her time as a family planning adviser in the 1970s. She told reporters: "I had to travel alone going door to door and these mullahs would tell people to beat me up with a stick. They got me sacked because I was unmarried." She and other women were standing for election in 2013 to show that women could have a say in their own future and could get elected, despite the threats.

Nationalism

Religious fundamentalism is not the only factor in campaigns against contraception. Nationalism, too, can come into play. Two examples are from the former Soviet bloc in Eastern Europe. In Romania under Nicolae Ceausescu, contraception and abortion were banned in order to force women to have babies they often could not feed, clothe or house. Ceausescu announced: "The foetus is the socialist property of the whole society. Giving birth is a patriotic duty… Those who refuse to have children are deserters." The result was great misery, with the highest maternal mortality rates in Europe, and 87% of the deaths were the result of dangerous abortions. Large numbers of babies and children were abandoned in State orphanages, which were filthy and hugely overcrowded, and care was rudimentary at best. A movement arose among childless couples in western countries to adopt these "orphans" (although their parents were often still alive). Many of the children suffered permanent illness and disability as a result of the physical and emotional neglect they had suffered.

The other example was the former Soviet Union, where contraceptives were almost impossible to get but abortions were freely offered at government clinics, and frequent abortions were the only way for most women to prevent unwanted births. These operations were often done without anaesthetic, a form of torture that seemed to be a punishment for not producing a baby for the Motherland. The Soviets had suffered huge losses of both soldiers and civilians in the Second World War and were trying to encourage large families through withholding contraception, a "childless" tax, and medals and rewards for Hero Mothers who had large families. The policy simply did not work in towns and cities because women were unable to look after babies and children while doing their obligatory full-time jobs, and living in overcrowded shared flats. They were very unwilling to leave children in the State nurseries, which, apart from those catering for the elite, were inadequate and even dangerous.

There are countries where the population is declining, including probably modern Russia – although the statistics on this have been questioned. The most important cause of declining population numbers is out-migration, in situations where the prospects for younger people are simply better elsewhere. Their own children will probably be born in other countries. This applies mainly in Eastern and Southern Europe, with migration to Western Europe, together with Cuba and Puerto Rico both losing people to the US. By 2030 it is predicted that falling numbers will also apply to China, Japan, Thailand, Italy, Greece and Spain, based on current fertility and migration levels.

Putting pressure on people to have more children, when they know they cannot care for them, simply does not work but merely produces misery. In western Europe between the two world wars, after the huge losses of men during the First World War, many governments had pro-natalist policies which included State subsidies for extra babies. Yet with an economic depression, unemployment, poverty and poor housing, people could not afford to have many children and did whatever they could to avoid births. Birth rates fell rapidly, even though contraception at that time was far less good than today's (many relied on the withdrawal method) and abortion was illegal.

My own grandparents were caught up in this dilemma: they both worked for an institution which provided their food, but not their children's – they had to pay per child out of their meagre wages. When a "surprise" third child arrived he had to be kept secret, and hidden away when inspectors came. If people had sex outside marriage at that time, men were under no obligation to support any children that resulted. Women were literally "left holding the baby," as it was described, and subjected to the great shame of illegitimacy – hence the desperation to "get rid of it" and the high levels of extremely dangerous abortions or young women being forced to give up their babies for adoption.

In that situation it was the people who decided whether to have children, and governments that had to accept the outcome. In other situations, governments, religious fundamentalists and nationalist or sectarian movements are able to force people to have children through their public campaigns, opposition to family planning and, sometimes, personal threats. These, too, are driven by men who take little or no personal responsibility for looking after the extra children they help to create. In some cases they distort the truth about human bodies with outrageous fictions. Some Catholic organisations, for instance, misrepresent contraceptives as "really" abortion, or claim dangers from terminations ("abortion causes cancer") that do not exist. Meanwhile some ultra-conservatives in the United States openly justify rape, and enforced childbirth if that is the result. Some have made startling claims that women "raped easy" and would not resist but only call it rape the next morning, and that in any case it could not have been rape if the woman became pregnant. Babies that resulted from a rape would be "God's gifts". Or should that be "My God's punishment on you"?

"Family planning is a pro-life cause"

If religious fundamentalists and nationalists would only devote their attention to the real welfare of their communities, including the care and upbringing of children, and if they insisted on the responsibilities of men, there might be some justification for their wanting more children. If only they would campaign for a genuinely moral approach, and against exploitative and violent behaviour in relationships, they might acquire moral credibility. A non-fundamentalist Catholic priest quoted by the journalist Chris Hedges has it about right:"Faith always starts with oneself. It means an overriding sense of responsibility for the universe, making sure that universe is left in good hands…"

It is important to remember that the fundamentalists do not represent mainstream religious approaches, although they often claim to do so. Nor are all conservatives necessarily on the wrong side. Many faith-based organisations are working quietly but effectively to promote safe sex, contraception, and sometimes abortion as well. Meanwhile, let us conclude with the comment of a US evangelical Christian and conservative columnist, Michael

Gerson, who saw this work on the ground in rural areas of the Democratic Republic of Congo. Speaking at a conference in 2013 he said: "[Family planning] is often a controversial topic here in [Washington] DC, but it shouldn't be. When births are spaced more than 24 months apart, both mothers and children are dramatically more likely to survive. In cases like this, family planning is a pro-life cause, and everyone should support it."

Resources

Michelle Goldberg, "The Great Population Panic" in *The Means of Reproduction: Sex, Power and the Future of the World* (Penguin Press, New York, 2009).

Mark Steyn, *America Alone: The End of the World As We Know* It (Regnery Publishing, Washington DC, 2006).

Pat Buchanan, *The Death of the West: How Dying Populations and Immigrant Invasions Imperil Our Country and Civilization* (St Martin's Press, New York, 2002).

Soldaten: On Fighting, Killing and Dying, by Sonke Neitzel and Harald Welzer (Simon & Schuster, 2013).

TV Channel Five (UK), "Children of the Master Race," 21 November 2013.

Gloria Steinem, article in *Speak Out Against the New Right,* edited by Herbert F.Vetter (Boston: Beacon Press, 1982).

Jonathan V Last, *What to Expect When No-one's Expecting* (Encounter Books, 2013).

GISA: Global Interfaith and Secular Alliance, convened by Catholics for Choice and the Asian-Pacific Resource & Research Centre for Women.

Association for Women's Rights in Development (AWID): papers on fundamentalism: "New Insights on Religious Fundamentalisms, Research Highlights," September 2009, and "Exposed: Ten Myths About Religious Fundamentalisms," by Cassandra Balchin, November 2008.

Dr Mehtab S Karim, "Population Bomb", *The News*, Pakistan, 6 April 201.

Ziba Mir-Hosseini   and others (eds): *"Gender and Equality in Muslim Family Law: Justice and Ethics in the Islamic Legal Tradition"*, IB Tauris, London, 2013.

"How the Taliban undermined community healthcare in Swat, Pakistan," by Iftikhar Ud Din and others, *British Medical Journal, 21 March 2012.*

Sneha Barot, "A Common Cause: Faith-Based Organizations and Promoting Access to Family Planning in the Developing World," *Guttmacher Policy Review,* Fall 2013, Volume 16, Number 4.

Chapter four

DORIAN GRAY LIVES!
The fear of an "ageing society"

In the richer countries there are regular, loud claims that they are in an "ageing society" and this is often used to justify claims that everybody must have more children. It conjures up for me Oscar Wilde's story, "The Picture of Dorian Gray". A beautiful young man is haunted by his own portrait, even though it is hidden away in the attic. This picture ages rapidly and within days it moves to a hideous old age, decay and death, revealing his own corruption and his hideous future. "What the worm was to the corpse, his sins would be to the painted image on the canvas. They would mar its beauty and eat away its grace. They would defile it and make it shameful. And yet the thing would live on. It would be always alive." In the end the picture does show him dead. "Suddenly, time stopped for him. Yes, that blind, slow-breathing thing crawled no more, and horrible thoughts, time being dead, raced nimbly on in front, and dragged a hideous future from its grave, and showed it to him. He stared at it. Its very horror made him stone."

This is one of the very few stories ever written that, in an age-obsessed world, directly addresses our desperate longing to hold on to our youth, and our fear of getting old. I would have to look back at my own teenage self to confess that I too, as a young person, wondered what those grey-looking old people were for, and even had the fleeting thought that they might as well die soon. Now I am older, I finally understand what older people are for...

Dorian Gray syndrome seems to lie behind much of the discussion among politicians and demographers about the "ageing society" and how awful that must be (especially as they are themselves approaching this category, or are already there). The solution they put forward, all too often, is: more babies! Now! Get breeding, quick... never mind if some die before they even start working for us, we'll just get more. Make sure those women give us young people to provide more cheap labour, so there will be plenty of them to look after us oldies and keep us alive and healthy as long as possible. Why should we care about their future? We will be dead!

There are many other countries where panic is apparently rising about their supposedly "ageing society", fostered strangely by the United Nations and its agencies. A report from the UN children's agency Unicef in 2012 claims: "The global old-age dependency rate will accelerate markedly, almost tripling from 12% in 2010 to around 32% in 2070." Some agencies define "old" as over 60: a country may officially become "an ageing society" when people of 60 years of age or older account for 10% of the total population, according to current UN definitions. Unicef defines it as 65 and above, but also assumes that older people are inevitably dependent on younger ones. There is no subtlety here, no recognition of older people's role in the community as a whole.

"Old age dependency" is an article of faith for Unicef and other agencies, and older people are wicked consumers of "essential resources" that should be going to more and more children. Perhaps they will be calling older people witches next, with special reference to those pesky women who will continue to live longer than men. So the witch must die.

Consider for example this pronouncement from a leading Chinese official, Lou Jiwei. "The Chinese population is aging and labor costs are increasing. Without due measures, China will lose its edge over other countries." Professor Cai Fang, director of the Institute of Population and Labor Economics, has argued that, as a result of its "one child" policy, China was losing its "demographic dividends" as ageing had accelerated and the dependency ratio (the number of children and the elderly compared to working-age adults) had stopped declining in 2011. His solution: to "get" more children – disregarding the fact that this would add further to the dependency ratio for at least another 16 years.

In the real world, older people have a crucial role in supporting those who really are dependent, often at great cost to themselves. Many are working, earning money or helping the younger members of the family or community. They may be caring for others, many of them bringing up grandchildren when parents work elsewhere, die or become sick and disabled. Many older people do unpaid voluntary work in the community. In the process, they are saving huge amounts of money in care costs that would otherwise fall to local and national governments, and they are keeping alive people who would otherwise die. Perhaps Unicef disapproves of older people who feed and look after children? In Britain alone, research by Carers UK shows the economic value of work by carers is a massive £119 billion a year, and growing rapidly. This is bigger than the total budget of the National Health Service. If you are working long hours to care unpaid for a dependent person, is it not an insult to have yourself described as a dependent?

There are indeed massive changes in the age structure of populations almost everywhere in the world, but the biggest change of all is in the younger age groups in the poorer countries, while a much smaller trend is more adults living beyond 60 or 65 in the richer ones. Both of these trends are the result of the same phenomenon: successful campaigns to improve people's health and survival rates. They are a necessary element in the transition from many births and many deaths to a greatly reduced mortality for everyone, in practically all countries. You would find it hard to find a demographer or politician who wanted to bring back population control by death as an instrument of policy – therefore they have to accept that there will be imbalances in the age structure if we hope to move towards a stable and balanced population, as well as a healthier one. Panic attacks over the "ageing society" and "dependency ratios" merely obstruct the move towards this goal.

There is something seriously wrong with the numbers where people are counted as "economically productive" or "dependents" based purely on their age. The reality is far more complex. Let us remember that many older people – and children too – contribute to household incomes. At the same time there are increasing numbers of sick and disabled people who survive childhood, especially in poor regions and countries, to become dependent on others while of "working age" – not through their choice but often because of discrimination in their own societies, and lack of the health care and equipment available in richer countries. Many able-bodied young people, who should be entering the workforce and helping to maintain themselves and their families, also remain economically dependent because of enormously high levels of unemployment. The number of jobs, and the availability of land and other assets, is far below the numbers entering what should be a "working age".

Getting younger every day

An excellent demolition of the notion of an "ageing population" as some kind of problem is offered by Jeroen Spijker and John MacInnes, who looked in detail at the situation in Britain. They argued that the conventional "old age dependency ratio" is a poor measure of real dependency:

"The population of 2009, despite being much older as measured by years lived, was nevertheless younger than that of 1900 in terms of years left. This is crucial, because many behaviours and attitudes (including those related to health) are more strongly linked to remaining life expectancy than to age … rising life expectancy makes these older people 'younger', healthier, and fitter than their peers in earlier cohorts."

For Spijker and MacInnes, the cut-off point is 15 years or less of life expectancy. Most acute medical care costs, they add, occur in the final months of life, and the age at which these months occur has little relevance. So a disadvantaged young person who cannot survive long is really "older" than someone with many more years on the clock who enjoys good health.

Spijker and MacInnes also have some challenging thoughts on the so-called "working age" population, where there have been huge changes in recent years. In countries with longer life expectancy, numbers of pensioners have been kept down by raising the age at which people can claim. Young people now start working much later, because of the growth of higher education, while many older workers either retire earlier or later than a fixed age. Meanwhile, greater sex equality and dual career families have added five million women workers to the British labour market over the past 50 years. "If we count people who are not employed, for whatever reason, as dependent, we find that there are more dependants of working age (9.5 million) than there are older people who do not work."

These are powerful trends, moving in opposite directions and making nonsense of the old assumptions about "working age". "We calculated what we call the real elderly dependency ratio as the sum of men and women with a remaining life expectancy ≤15 years [15 years or less] divided by the number of people in employment. When we use this as a measure, dependency has fallen by one third over the past four decades." So much for the panic over increased dependency through "ageing".

The rates are very variable among the richer countries. The United States has a lower ratio than the UK, while in Germany and Italy the real elderly dependency ratio has been almost flat for two decades. Only Japan, which is unusual in having a combination of relatively low birth rates with very little immigration or women in the labour force, has seen its ratio rise rapidly.

Call yourself a dependant?

In poorer countries and regions the real dependency issue is the "youth bulge", where survival rates of children have improved greatly while births remained at a high level. Many if not most of the young people in this cohort are forced to be dependent on others while scraping a half-living in bits of casual work, entering sex work with all its dangers and abuses, or turning to crime, gangs and terrorist organisations to survive. Unemployed young people are moving in huge numbers to towns and cities that are already massively overcrowded. Some of them face death as they cross oceans or climb frontier fences to a perhaps illusory promised land in a richer country. If anything, this generation will face even worse problems as more and more children swell the ranks of the supposedly "working-aged" – young people for whom there is no work and no livelihood.

The best way to help the armies of unemployed young people, and the children coming up behind them, would be to help women reduce the numbers of babies being born who, in around 15 years' time, will compete with and perhaps undercut them in the battle for jobs, land, food, water, education, housing, health care and even survival itself.

The consequences of all this are apparent in most of the "youth bulge" countries. The situation in Mexico, for example, is described by Pedro Salazar Ugarte, writing in the *Boston Review* about the violence and instability afflicting his country, despite its being one of the fastest-growing economies: "Mexico … may take off or it may collapse. And I do not exaggerate or mean this rhetorically. Never before has Mexico had so many young people: nearly 30 million men and women aged 15–29, representing 26.4% of the country's population. They are what we call in Mexico the "demographic bonus," at first considered a great opportunity to enhance the country's growth and development, and now a threat to its existence. Millions of them have been excluded from these key social institutions: learning and work. Young men and women, Mexico's future, are being left without futures of their own… If Mexico does not guarantee its young people a fair chance at success, it can expect a violent future."

This is also the conclusion that David Kilcullen comes to in his survey of urban unrest in many rapidly growing coastal cities, especially in the developing world. "A megacity under stress can offer opportunities for conflict entrepreneurs (gang leaders, crime bosses or militant extremists) to control populations, provided they create a predictable rule set that makes people feel safe in the face of instability … whether people like the group

or not, and regardless of the content of those rules. Eventually
… it may gain the loyalty and support of the local population."
Although he describes this in fairly neutral terms, we are talking
about organisations which seek to take over control of areas by
means of protection and extortion rackets: pay our percentage,
sell our drugs, and above all keep quiet about what you know.
Otherwise you or your family members risk death, and your
family's livelihood could be destroyed.

This is a system of organised terror that, once entrenched,
is very hard for a democratic government to control. Italy's
Mafia and 'Ndrangheta organisations are well-known examples.
They grew up over centuries of shifting colonial conquest and
occupation, with weak local governments, and are bigger than
ever now with their shift to drug dealing, people trafficking,
prostitution and crime generally, which now extends worldwide.
There are many other criminal gangs in other countries which
have national and international reach, starting in different
local areas that all had the common feature of a lack of central
authority, and no alternative livelihood for many young people.
The pirates based in lawless Somalia are just one of the better-
known examples.

Another example of this is urban Kenya, where the National
Crime Research Centre has identified at least 46 criminal gangs,
some of them as violent as the al-Shabaab group that attacked
the Westgate shopping centre in Nairobi. These gangs have come
to dominate the city's shanty towns, which account for more
than 60% of Nairobi's population. Kilcullen argues that with an
expected three billion new urban-dwellers expected to arrive in
the megacities by the middle of this century, the disruption by
gangs and crime bosses could dwarf the threat of terrorism from
groups like Da'esh (ISIS) or al-Shabaab. Finding community

solutions to these problems, he adds, could be impossible "when the community is under threat and someone is shooting at you".

The situation arises not only from the sheer numbers, but also of course from the extreme inequality of opportunity and wealth, which is a characteristic of most developing countries, especially those with the highest economic growth rates. Nigeria is another example of these two factors coming together: its 5.7% fertility rate is already acting as a fierce brake on development in spite of the wealth generated by oil production, which ends up in the hands of a privileged few. Professor Oladapo Ladipo explains that it is hard to grow the economy because of the high dependency, especially of children, and the consequences for their cash-starved parents. "Because you are spending all of your money just trying to help these dependents survive… then you do not have any money left over to invest in economic activities, business, and more education."

A universal poverty can also spark tragedy if there are disproportionate numbers of landless and unemployed young people. Journalists reporting on the sudden outbreak of sectarian violence between Christians and Muslims in the Central African Republic have reported that young men who suddenly got access to a Kalashnikov rifle would use it to threaten or kill their neighbours and seize their homes, land and whatever possessions they had. It is a pattern that has been seen in all too many countries around the world.

New definitions: dependency revisited

Demographers are finding it hard to include all these considerations in their definition of dependency. They define it simply as "ageing", largely because that is easy to measure – at least in countries that have reasonable records of births and deaths. Unfortunately, this easy route presents a badly distorted picture of who in the population is economically productive, and who is really a dependent. It fails to count adults of working age who are forced to be dependent on others. To bring this waste of human talent and human energy into the statistics would transform population policies around the world.

So this is my suggestion: use selective sampling alongside the (sometimes unreliable) national statistics to more accurately define dependency ratios. The work would involve judgements of how to allocate individuals and families living complex lives and with varying degrees of support and dependency, but in poor communities these relationships, complicated as they are, need to be better understood. The categories I suggest would be:

Economically active

• *Employed and self-employed*
This category would include all those working in regular jobs, full- or part-time, or running a regular business with assets (for example a shop or trading operation).
• *Farmers and agricultural workers*
Farmers (including subsistence farmers) would be prominent in this group, with women playing a particularly important role. A large part of their income is in kind rather than money, in the form of food in particular, but most of them are also able to earn a little cash, which is essential for sending children to school, clothing, transport, medical care and other items.
• *Casual workers*
This would particularly cover the huge numbers of people, especially in poor countries, who have no land of their own and no regular jobs or business, but are essential earners nonetheless.

They could be running micro-enterprises in street trading, labouring, dressmaking or other casual work, or for huge numbers of women there is sex work. In many cases these would be the people bringing in the cash on which whole families would have to survive.

• *Retired and self-sufficient*

These would be people over retirement age who are not financially dependent on family members. Some would still be earning, many have their own pension or other income and are able to meet their own needs. They may also give financial or practical help to younger family members, and many contribute to society as unpaid volunteers.

• *Essential carers*

This is the group of people who may not be economically active in cash terms, but who make a crucial contribution to families, society as a whole, and the economy. They may be assisting working family members and others, or they may provide essential care for ill and disabled people, mainly in their own families.

Huge numbers of older people, previously considered to be "dependants", would come into this category. In developing countries with no social services, pensions or benefits system, many older people – mainly women – would be keeping others going, including for example looking after the children of wage-earners, or providing them with food and other essentials. There is usually no cash payment involved.

Some kind of estimate of the value of this work would be extremely useful, even though exact numbers may be hard to come by. In Britain, a report from the insurer RIAS in 2012 calculated that 5.8 million grandparents were regularly looking after children, providing a cash saving in childcare of nearly £11 billion a year. In relative terms the value is likely to be even higher in poorer countries, particularly in countries like the Philippines with high out-migration, where wage earners may have to move to other countries to support their family and leave their children behind with other relatives.

Economic dependants

• *Dependent children:* children up to the age of 15, but with a reduction to reflect the extent to which children are economically active. High proportions of children, especially in developing countries, are contributing financially to their families or simply scraping a living on their own – this obviously applies to abandoned or orphaned street children, but it also involves the legions of children living with their own families who are earning, often in domestic service, manufacturing, street selling and begging. There is also a very high level of contribution by children in farming and labouring families in rural areas. Children also very often look after younger brothers and sisters.

• *Dependent adults unable to work:* these would of course include many older people, but only if they are true dependents rather than classified on the basis of age alone. There would also be sick and disabled people, who would of course include "working-age" adults, and this would help to draw attention to the extremely high level of disability in many poorer countries resulting from malnutrition and preventable disease. It also arises from injuries suffered by mothers and babies at birth, the result of unintended, closely spaced pregnancies, inadequate nutrition and poor health systems.

•*Dependent unemployed:* a key dependency element which would describe the enormous numbers of young people who are not needed to work within the family, and cannot find a job or other livelihood elsewhere. This category would highlight the problem of unemployment among the "youth bulge", and help to focus the attention of politicians on the issue of how their people need to live rather than merely existing. This category is in fact quite difficult to measure: some kind of sample survey would be needed to assess the numbers of truly unemployed and unproductive people. There is often no absolute dividing line − unemployed people may turn to occasional casual work or street trading when they can, or in desperation may turn to drug dealing, sex work and theft to relieve their dependent or destitute state.

•*Criminals as dependants in the "grey economy":* It could be argued that theft, dealing in drugs and other anti-social activity is much worse than being a "dependant" in that it actively exploits other people, may impoverish or kill them, and has the worst effect on the poorest people. It is obviously related to the very high unemployment rates. Also in this category would be the street gangs and terror networks.

In modern economic and political terms, what is not measured in a country is not valued, or even noticed. By revising our counting of "economically active" and "dependent" people within a population we can provide a basis for much more realistic policies. Obviously − unlike age categories − the dividing lines between the different groups I am suggesting are uncertain: for example, someone may be unemployed but occasionally earn a bit of money. Definitions would have to be worked on, and perhaps arbitrary distinctions made. This exercise would be well worth it, however, because it would highlight the real contributors and dependants within a population as a whole, and provide the background for more realistic policies. These would have to include a new focus on the numbers of babies being born, the welfare of women as well as men, the value of unpaid work, and the importance of health and welfare in reducing dependency. It leads on to an even bigger question of how we define gross domestic product (GDP) and even economic growth and development as a whole, because of the importance of non-cash contributions to the welfare of individuals and society.

The second demographic dividend

It is time to get over the moral panic about the prospect of fewer babies and more older people, which some have even called a "demographic winter". This panic is hugely overstated even for richer countries, which have had rapid increases in life expectancy. This may not continue: there are many indications that our age span may fall if predictions are right about the increasing resistance of bacteria to life-saving antibiotics, the effects of unhealthy diets and lack of exercise, obesity and a rapid increase in Type 2 diabetes. In the UK, for instance, three million people already have Type 2 diabetes and a third of the population are pre-diabetic.

The exaggerated warnings of a supposedly "ageing population" are also being applied to areas where there is little or no sign of this happening: sub-Saharan Africa, which has the lowest percentage of older people in the world, and Latin America where numbers are also low and, although growing, are doing so only very slowly. In reality, as Elizabeth Leahy Madsen has pointed out, the process of what she describes as "population maturity" is slow, and for most countries any significant extension of life expectancy remains on the distant horizon. She argues that there is plenty of time to rethink what it could mean when and if it really does happen. It could mean a boost, and not a threat, to economic development and growth.

The "second demographic dividend" from increased life expectancy arises from the contributions made by older people who have had a long working life. They may continue to contribute themselves, and many have accumulated pension savings, money that is invested in the productive economy and provides large numbers of jobs for the younger generation.

While many richer countries are benefiting from this process, it does depend on there being enough money around – including welfare benefits – and health systems which can keep people productive. Without this, a country might have significant numbers of older people but be unable to keep them fit and healthy. The main examples here are Russia, which has high rates of chronic illness and disability, and the United States, where many people cannot save enough to meet their needs in retirement, including medical treatment when they need it. In poor countries the relatively few people who do live into older age have generally not earned enough to save, and too often face real poverty. Traditionally, they would have been supported by younger family members but for some of them, these support systems are breaking down. This seems to be a particular issue in China. The solutions lie in tackling the welfare problems to ensure self-reliance and health for older people, not in worrying about their numbers.

Of course towards the end of their lives some older people in all countries do become dependent, and may eventually need help with their health and daily tasks. Governments in countries where this is a real issue need to come up with innovative schemes to match the "really old" with the increasing numbers of what has been called "young old" retired people, many of them on reasonable pensions, who have plenty of time and often many of the skills needed.

Many of those retirees already provide many hours of voluntary work for friends, family and the community at large, while others complain of not having enough to do. Perhaps they could be offered a form of partnership or co-operative scheme where they enrol as informal carers for others, and in return get a guarantee that if they then need informal care later on it will be there for them. Together with better help and support for full-time family carers and a good backup service for those with the most acute needs, especially in their own homes, the quality and effectiveness of care can be hugely improved compared to what is on offer at present. New Zealand is a leader in developing a comprehensive strategy for end of life and palliative care, based on advance care plans which are drawn up in consultation with patients, backed by sophisticated communication systems and training for health practitioners who work in end-of-life care.

A mature and balanced population?
A healthy population will have a balance of different ages, together with systems for supporting those who really need it – children, the unemployed, and people with severe illness or disabilities. As people become healthier, and death rates at all ages decline, there will inevitably be more individuals living longer. This is a symptom of success, not failure. We all, as individuals, are getting older from the day we are born until the day we die, and to see this as some kind of disaster is a distortion of our human aspirations as well as our wellbeing as a society.

So let the demographers and politicians celebrate age as well as youth, seeing all of us as an essential resource. Can we finally ditch the fearful spectre of an "ageing society" and see it instead as our final rejection of premature death as a limiter of population? An increasing average age of the population is natural and inevitable as soon as fertility rates begin to fall. From an economic perspective, ageing that happens early in the demographic transition is a good thing because it signals that the age structure is becoming more balanced, the dependency ratio is falling, and a larger percentage of the population is composed of working-age people who can generate income.

The "ageing" scare? Dorian Gray still lives, it seems. It is time to lay him quietly to rest. RIP.

Resources

Jack A Goldstone et al, eds, "Political Demography: How Population Changes are Reshaping International Security and National Politics (Paradigm and Pluto Press, 2012).

David Kilcullen, "Out of the Mountains: The coming age of the urban guerrilla," (Hurst, 2013).

Elizabeth Leahy Madsen, "For Fast-Growing Countries, Should Aging Be A Concern? Planning for the Second Demographic Dividend" The Wilson Centre website, 10 September 2013.

Jeroen Spijker and John MacInnes, "Population ageing: the timebomb that isn't?" British Medical Journal, 12 November 2013.

Chapter five

A MODERN INQUISITION?
The Catholic hierarchy: a war on women's choices

"Though I speak with the tongues of men and of angels, and have not charity, I am become as sounding brass, or a tinkling cymbal."

"And though I have the gift of prophecy, and understand all mysteries, and all knowledge; and though I have all faith, so that I could remove mountains, and have no charity, I am nothing."

(1ˢᵗ letter from St Paul to the Corinthians, 13: 1-2. King James Bible, Cambridge edition)

Does the Catholic hierarchy have the gift of charity? Many critics would say they put dogma first – seeking perhaps to remove mountains with it – while closing their ears to the needs of the people. In the western Catholic tradition they are all celibate males, they observe, constantly obsessed with women's bodies while ignorant of how women really live their lives. Even more important, perhaps, they have never had children (not legally, anyway) and do not live in families, so have no personal experience of what this really means, even though they preach long and loud about what "the family" should be.

One of my favourite stories is from Boccaccio's *Decameron*. Some Catholic priests were trying to convert a Jewish man to their religion and thought they were doing splendidly until he told them he was so impressed by their faith that he was going to make a pilgrimage to Rome. They were horrified: one look at the corruption and excesses of the Vatican at that time and their convert would run a mile. He returned, full of enthusiasm and determined to be baptised. Why? He explained: if a Church is vibrant enough to thrive in the hearts of the people in spite of all that happens in Rome, it must indeed be close to God.

I am reminded of this story as I look at the Catholic hierarchy's campaign to promote Catholic births, and particularly its campaign to stop people using contraception and abortion. In the name of a "pro-life" mission, and contrary to the traditions of the Church in past ages, for the last century and a half they have made this their number one priority, the subject of endless decrees and dogmas, and with greater priority for their attention than the genuine life issues such as capital punishment, war or murder. In the 1930 document *Casti Connubii (On Chaste Wedlock)* the then Pope, Pius XI, declared artificial contraception to be "intrinsically evil," something that could never be permitted for any reason. Even murder is not considered by the Church to be in this category. The hierarchy have even, at times, traded a tolerance for extreme cruelty in return for governments' adherence to their "Life" crusade. Catholic priests have been implicated recently in justifying or even promoting torture and murder in Argentina and Rwanda, for example, in return for greater political commitment to their campaigns against contraception and abortion.

This obsession with stopping women from planning their pregnancies is all the more bizarre because virtually all the church's members ignore the hierarchy's teachings on family choice if they can, that is, if contraceptives are available. In

Spain and Italy, both of them strongly Catholic, birth rates have dropped dramatically to near-replacement levels. In the United States, the Guttmacher Institute reported in 2011 that 87% of Catholic women at risk of unplanned pregnancy were using contraceptives, barely below the national average of 88%. Among women of reproductive age who had ever had sex, 98% of Catholic women had used contraceptives compared to 99% of all women. So the number of Catholics obeying their Church's teachings against artificial contraception is minimal – as low as one in a hundred. It is likely that the findings would be similar in other countries provided there was easy access to family planning and the Church had not managed to prevent that through pressure on governments.

It has been suggested that the hierarchy's extreme vehemence on this issue is precisely because of their failure to enforce their teachings among their own members. What this means in practice is that in countries where they have overwhelming political power – including Ireland, the Philippines, and much of Latin America – they are all the more determined to block people's access to contraceptive services, and especially legal and safe abortion, by putting pressure on governments to pass legislation or issue decrees.

Alongside relentless pressure on governments, they can also use their monopoly provision of health services in many parts of the developing world to make sure that people cannot get contraception or safe abortions. For millions of the poorest people around the world, health provision is either a Catholic "mission" hospital or clinic, or nothing at all. Even for the wealthy elite, in many developing countries the main Catholic hospital is often the best (and most expensive) available to them. That will certainly not be offering family planning services or safe terminations, although if people can afford it they will have access to clinics elsewhere.

Why does the Catholic Church have such a powerful influence on the issue of choice about childbirth? It is partly because of its enormous membership in so many countries of the world. This is compounded by its near-monopoly on medical services in many of the poorest areas. Even more important, however, is the enormous amount of "diplomatic" and lobbying work undertaken at the United Nations, international conferences, and with many individual governments to block people's access to contraception and safe abortion, as we shall see in Chapter 7.

Where did it all go wrong?

For such a high-profile element of the Catholic Church's teachings and dogma, you might assume that this has been an article of faith either from Jesus's teachings or starting with the very early Church. This is not so.

The Catholic theologian Christine Gudorf has pointed out that Christianity evolved in a world in which contraception and abortion were known about, and certainly used. Egyptians, Jews, Greeks and Romans are known to have used pessaries, potions and condoms as well as *coitus interruptus* (the man withdrawing before ejaculation) while abortion also seems to have been widespread. Medieval Islamic physicians listed 196 contraceptive substances. Vaginal sponges and douches were often used. A Greek legend described a female condom made of a goat's bladder. The same was true of abortion: two thousand years ago a wild fennel growing all around the Mediterranean area, which was used to terminate pregnancy, was used so extensively that it became extinct.

However the most important method of limiting family size was, sadly, infanticide – often recorded as "smothering" or "rolling over", or deaths recorded as "stillbirths" when in fact the babies died after birth. Unwanted babies were deliberately killed, neglected, or abandoned with little or no food or clothing. Of the Church's response, Gudorf writes: "The primary pastoral battles in the first millennium were around infanticide, the banning of which undoubtedly raised the incidence of abandonment."

Abandonment meant babies left to die of hunger, thirst and cold, abandoned in wild areas to be killed by animal predators, or left in the road for anybody to take. If these babies survived this would often mean lifelong slavery or abuse, living lives of great suffering and perhaps an early death. To ease the crisis and the human agony – of the mothers as well as the children – the Church in the middle ages encouraged people to offer babies they could not care for to foundling hospitals or to the Church, to be brought up as celibate nuns and monks who would serve the Church all their lives. Although they were denied a family life, this was at least better than the alternative. It was also an important source of support for the Church itself.

The history of the Church's teachings on contraception and abortion up to the 19th century shows absolutely no consistency on these issues. No proclamations against it have been found in any biblical texts, and extensive research has failed to find them in the history of the early Church either. The first pontifical intervention found was in 1484, when Europe was starting to recover from the massive epidemic known as the Black Death, which killed millions. Inquisitor Kramer urged Pope Innocent VIII to act against sorcerers who, he claimed, "hinder men from performing the sexual act and women from conceiving." Church witch-hunts and the killing of old women as "witches" probably had much to do with church fears that they were helping women avoid childbirth. Clearly, contraception was being practised by believers throughout Church history. Male condoms, which had been made out of a wide variety of natural materials including animal skins, were mass-produced from the 19th century with the use of rubber, and became much more widely used.

Even now, the Church allows and even promotes supposedly "natural" birth control, otherwise known as the rhythm method, which calculates the recommended times for sex when the woman is least likely to be fertile. The main problem with it is that it can be quite stressful, requires a level of communication between couples that few can achieve, and is fairly ineffective, although modern developments with computer and mobile phone apps have improved it. As the observer HL Mencken has written: "It is now quite lawful for a Catholic woman to avoid pregnancy by resort to mathematics, though she is still forbidden to resort to physics or chemistry." Nobody could accuse the Church of a logical consistency.

Daniel Maguire, who has written extensively on the development of Church dogma on abortion in particular, has concluded that there was never a single teaching: "The Roman Catholic position on abortion is pluralistic. It has a strong 'pro-choice' tradition and a conservative anti-choice tradition. Neither is official and neither is more Catholic than the other." Indeed, the present dogma depends not on any Catholic tradition but on a modern scientific understanding of pregnancy and childbirth. Until very recently, little was known about how embryos and foetuses developed before birth. It was even imagined that a man's sperm were little "homunculi" or miniature people (for this reason male masturbation was sometimes called homicide). The equal role of the woman's eggs was not known and the development of the fertilised egg into a zygote, an embryo and then a foetus was also not understood. For this reason life or "ensoulment" was generally believed to start many weeks after conception, generally at the "quickening" when the woman could feel the foetus moving, usually early in the fifth month of pregnancy. The woman was then the vessel for the future child, which had developed fully formed out of the man's sperm.

The Church's traditional teachings about sex and childbirth were generally based on a view of women as intrinsically inferior and a source of temptation that men should resist. It is an approach that even the most conservative man in the hierarchy would blush to acknowledge today, although it must remain deep in their collective subconscious. As Daniel Maguire points out, "A culture that looks on women as sources of evil like Pandora and Eve is going to have trouble justifying [men] having sex with them." St Augustine said that, were it not for reproduction, there would be no use for women at all. Some other early Church writers argued that women were like animals in that we lack reason, and only possess the image of God through connection to men. The feminist theologian Christine Gudorf points out that the Church has rejected this nonsense about women but "continues to teach most of the sexual moral code which was founded upon such thinking".

On the question of abortion, little was said specifically by the Church authorities until the 15th century and, even then, many theologians justified it in particular cases which included the life and welfare of the mother. There is even a Catholic saint, a Florentine archbishop of the 15th century called St Antoninus, who argued that early abortions were not murder because the foetus was not yet human. Influential writers of the 16th century and later went on to develop this view. The saint's namesake,

Antoninus of Corduba, wrote that the health as well as the life of the mother were more important than continuing a risky pregnancy. Perhaps we should nominate the two St Antoninuses as the official patron saints of World Contraceptive Day.

Even now, there are many different views among Catholic theologians and scholars on whether abortion is permissible in cases where there is danger of death for the mother, where conception occurred through rape, or where the foetus has died in the womb or is known to have a life-threatening disability. They would be well aware that Catholic families – like all families – depend on the mother's key role if they are to thrive, and therefore Catholic children need their mother to survive. You would not think that these alternative views existed within the Church, however, if you listen only to the hierarchy in Rome.

A recent scandal in Ireland highlights the extreme bias in parts of the Catholic Church towards promoting births without concern for the future lives of the babies. A mass grave of babies and children was discovered, some of them in a septic tank, at the former Bon Secours children's home in Tuam, Galway in 2017. They had been taken from unmarried mothers, in an atmosphere of "shame" over many decades, which made it almost impossible for the women to keep their children. Some babies were sold, often to American families who had not been vetted as suitable parents, or even to men on their own who claimed they had a wife. Some of the babies had been allowed to die in childbirth or in infancy and either buried without proper records or simply discarded in the tank where there was human waste. Some babies, born with a disability, were allowed to starve to death. Meanwhile many of the women were made to work without pay in Church-run laundries, continually told that they were wicked and sinful. No attempt was made to locate, and work with, the fathers, or to call them sinful for having sex outside marriage. Although this and similar homes have now been closed, it is estimated that 6,000 babies died in similar Church-run homes throughout Ireland.

"Infallible" Pius and the Life dogma

The Catholic hierarchy's implacable – one might even say fanatical – opposition to contraception and abortion originates as late as the end of the 19th century, when some modern methods were just beginning to become available. This opposition was reinforced in the 20th century, probably as a reaction to the improvements in those methods, and the easier access to them for women and couples who wanted to make their own choices.

The dogma is closely tied up with the notion of authority in the Church – exclusively male of course – and especially with the surprisingly recent idea of the Pope's "infallibility". "In every instance where the pope intervenes the bishops are obliged to obey and submit to his decisions." It was a radical reversal of centuries of Catholic Church history.

His "direct sovereignty over the entire Church" dates back to 1870 when Pius IX was faced with the conquest of the Papal States by the forces fighting for a unified Italy. He was also fighting a big expansion of the competing Protestant churches, as well as the secular revolutionary spirit epitomised by the French Revolution and 19th century popular movements for democracy and nationalism in Europe and worldwide.

With defeat on the battlefield by Garibaldi's unifying forces, Pius IX lost the historic secular powers that the Vatican had possessed to enforce authority in its own States through the arrest, imprisonment and even execution of opponents. It is telling perhaps that the last execution of a citizen of the Papal

States took place just six weeks before the formal introduction of the dogma of papal infallibility. It has been suggested that Pius was seeking a new absolute power over spiritual and doctrinal matters in the Church as a substitute for the lost power of life and death over his citizens. He was also under intense criticism from the popular press and from opinion within the Church.

At the time, this new dogma of papal infallibility was strongly opposed by many in the Church. Many bishops felt that Pius IX was insincere, malicious, perhaps insane, and using lies and trickery to force through a decision in his favour. One diarist wrote at the time: "Oh, this unfortunate pope. How much evil he has done!" The Catholic historian Franz Xavier Kraus wrote in his diary in 1900 that "Rome has locked the door leading to its only way out. There seems to be nothing left but for the whole papal system to break down." He was wrong.

The doctrine of infallibility was accepted by Church members as a whole, probably because it chimed with their own needs in a world full of turmoil. Mumford argues that "infallibility provides many believers with a great sense of religious security all through life, imparting stability and freedom from anxiety, relieving emotional pressure and softening the cruel blows of reality." In other words their personal happiness, both in this world and the next, depends on obedience to the Pope. He alone could provide a guarantee of their salvation after death. The well-connected Catholic writer John Bosco, who did much to promote the new doctrine of infallibility, even referred to the Pope as "God on earth". Pius IX has now been beatified by subsequent Popes, as has Bosco.

On the subject of contraception and abortion, major pronouncements were made in 1930 (with the encyclical *Casti connubii*), in 1951 (Pius XII's *Address to Midwives*), and 1958

(*Address to the Society of Haematology*). Finally in 1968 came the encyclical *Humanae Vitae* in which Pope Paul VI condemned practically every form of birth control as morally reprehensible. The *Encyclical* outlaws once and for all "any action which either before, at the moment of, or after sexual intercourse, is specifically intended to prevent procreation".

The sequence of events here shows just how fragile the dogma is. It could easily have gone in the opposite direction, if only Pope John XXIII had lived a little longer. He is thought to have taken that name, incidentally, after the 14th-century Pope John XXII who had condemned claims of his own "infallibility" as the work of the devil. When John XXIII set up his Papal Commission on Population and Birth in 1963, in response to the development of the contraceptive pill, it was a signal that the Church could change its position on birth planning in spite of the infallibility and authority principles. The Commission included leading Catholic theologians together with bishops and doctors, and even included five women.

In 1966 it reported, with strong majorities recommending change, that artificial birth control was not intrinsically evil and that Catholic couples should be allowed to decide for themselves about the methods to be employed. According to this report, use of contraceptives should be regarded as an extension of the already accepted rhythm or cycle method. Unfortunately, John XXIII had already died by the time the report was published. A minority report was dominated by the Polish cardinal Wojtyla (later Pope John Paul II) who insisted that any change of doctrine would be giving in to "the Protestants" and would mean conceding that the Holy Spirit had indeed been on the Protestant side. The new Pope Paul VI accepted this argument and turned the clock right back, using the minority report as justification, and issued *Humanae Vitae*.

Paul VI accepted the minority's argument that changing the dogma on contraception would undermine the authority of previous Church teachings. In effect the hierarchy is insisting on opposing contraception and abortion because they have done so previously, even if that was wrong. Mumford quotes Wojtyla, who wrote: "If it should be declared that contraception is not evil in itself, then we should have to concede frankly that the Holy Spirit had been on the side of the Protestant Churches … This would mean that the leaders of the Church, acting with extreme imprudence, had condemned thousands of innocent human acts, forbidding, under pain of eternal damnation, a practice which would now be sanctioned…"

Pope Paul VI followed his adoption of the minority report with a sweeping purge of the many Church officials and theologians who disagreed with it. The bishops of fourteen different countries had respectfully disagreed, and told their own Church members they could follow their own consciences. In many cases it was to cost them their jobs and career prospects, in a new (although thankfully less terrorising) Inquisition.

If this seems like the reaction of a dictator to any real or imagined threats to their authority, it reflects badly on a Church supposedly open to forgiveness and charity. Although the notion of papal infallibility is rarely used in a formal "*ex cathedra*" sense, it creates an aura of unquestionable authority on all decisions and announcements by successive Popes, even if they are different from their predecessors'. What is extraordinary is that among all the moral challenges in the world it is the issue of women, and their ability to decide on childbearing, which is seen by the authorities as the key test of the Pope's infallibility, and indeed of the Church's very authority on how we should all live our lives.

Looking for a way out

The Catholic Church, over the centuries, has shown that it can adjust to changing times, a changing economy, and new science, even though this is sometimes slow and reluctant. It no longer persecutes scientists such as Galileo, or forbids the payment of interest on loans, for example – previously seen as evil and strictly forbidden. The most notable recent example of major change is on the sexual abuse of children by priests, where the Church has turned from denial to condemnation, albeit only after a long and very painful battle by abuse victims and their supporters. The Church's official view of women has yet to be tackled: advocates of women's rights and needs are vocal within as well as outside the Church, but they are nowhere near strong enough to force a change of heart at the top.

Perhaps an all-male priesthood is just deeply resistant to women. The retired Pope Benedict XVI, when he was a Vatican official, even raised the spectre of the old fear of women, drafting an attack on the feminist movement which was issued as *A Letter to the Bishops of the Catholic Church on the Collaboration of Men and Women*. This claimed that feminist thought had destroyed "the family" and that it had induced women to see themselves as "the adversaries of men". As the philosopher Diana Maffia commented, the Letter fails to understand the women's movement but is a knee-jerk reaction to it:"It is not an invitation to dialogue, it attempts to enforce silence, undermine authority and make veiled threats."

Maguire sees this kind of thinking as a distortion of the Church's true message. He suggests that power in the Church is separated from ideas, which is a matter of real tragedy. "The Catholic tradition is more filled with good sense and flexibility than one would gather from its leaders" but popes and bishops, appointed by the existing hierarchy, are often bureaucratic careerists or natural conservatives who "often do not express the real treasures of wisdom that Catholicism has to offer to the world."

Is it possible that this wisdom could in the end prevail over the hierarchy in the matter of contraception and abortion? The purged Catholic theologian Hans Kung has concluded: "The only way to solve the problem of contraception is to solve the problem of infallibility." But there are Catholics who see a possibility of change based on a new focus on charity rather than authority, with a willingness to listen, especially to the poor, as preached by the current Pope, Francis. This remains to be seen: Francis is hated by many conservatives within the Catholic Church and one prominent English priest told *The Guardian*: "We can't wait for him to die. Whenever two of us meet, we talk about how awful he is." The atmosphere is poisonous, with Pope Francis telling the Italian newspaper *La Repubblica*: "Heads of the church have often been narcissists, flattered and thrilled by their courtiers. The court is the leprosy of the papacy."

There are entrenched attitudes and careers lined up behind the idea of papal authority, rather than the actual person of the Pope, and they have chosen the ban on modern contraception as their litmus test for loyalty. The Vatican's diplomatic missions around the world, especially at the United Nations, have for many years been devoted to undermining or blocking proposals to help women make our own decisions on sex and pregnancy. Bishops and cardinals in many countries have spent much of their time and effort lobbying governments to block choice. It is hard to see this edifice of opposition being dismantled any time soon. The most we might hope for is a reduction and softening of the campaign.

A new Inquisition?

It is the "Life" dogma, and the ferocious battle against contraception and abortion, that I compare to the medieval Inquisitions. The Catholic Church, alongside all the good it has done, has a shameful history of pursuing unbelievers, Protestants, "heretics", scientists and other dissidents, real or imagined. They included at one time their own Church members who had been forced to convert from Islam and Judaism, but were regarded as "unreliable" and prime targets for interrogation methods that would often lead to forced "confessions". With the book *Malleus Maleficarum* (*The Hammer of Witches*), elements of the Church also prompted and encouraged the medieval craze for witch-hunting, aimed mainly at women. One of the questions in this text was: "Whether Witches can Hebetate the Powers of Generation" and another was "That Witches who are Midwives in Various Ways Kill the Child Conceived in the Womb, and Procure an Abortion; or if they do not this Offer New-born Children to Devils."

There have been many different Inquisitions within the Catholic Church over the centuries, starting in the 12th century and continuing in some areas until the mid-19th century. The best known to us was in Spain, but in fact they covered many European countries and were vigorously pursued in the Spanish and Portuguese empires in Latin America, Africa and Asia. Suspects who were accused of "heretical" beliefs, or not conforming in some way, were tortured by priests, monks and others. Those convicted were handed over to civil authorities for imprisonment, banishment and execution, often by being burned alive. It was a campaign of terror: a 1578 handbook for inquisitors stated the objective as being "in order that others may become terrified and weaned away from the evils they would commit". After the Reformation, with some European countries becoming officially Protestant, the Church conducted violent campaigns forcing people back into the fold, in what was known as the Counter-Reformation. This involved not only individual persecution but also war (the French religious wars and the Thirty Years War) and massacres such as the St Bartholomew's Day Massacre in 1572 with a wave of Catholic mob violence against Protestants in Paris and other French cities. All this, sadly, was in the name of their Church's unquestionable authority, with charity nowhere to be seen.

With the Catholic hierarchy's modern Inquisition the main targets are now the women who will not or cannot conform to their authority, whether inside or outside the Church itself. There is obviously no physical torture done by priests themselves, and thankfully no murder. However the result is the same: the suffering and death of women and their children, enforced through the secular authorities by means of laws which the Church has demanded. Women are being exposed to the pain, disability and death which can result from too many pregnancies, the enormous risks of childbirth without good hygiene and medical care, and especially from illegal and botched abortions which are the result of desperate attempts to end unwanted pregnancies. Far too many of the babies born are also condemned to hunger and poverty, sometimes disability and an early death – especially if their mothers die, but also if there are more children than the family can support.

The inquisitorial approach also fosters and encourages verbal aggression, harassment and threats against women using family planning clinics, as well as the murder of doctors, arson, bomb attacks and sabotage of the clinics themselves. We will explore this further in Part Three. Some of those involved in this harassment are Catholics, others are not, but all are encouraged

and supported by Catholic "Life" dogma and generous support
and funding from the Church. A priest called Father Paul
Marx, who claims "contraception-sterilisation-abortion" is a
"worldwide plague", has set up Human Life International,
whose spokesman Don Treshman praised the sniper shooting of
a member of clinic staff in Canada as a "superb tactic". He also
started a fund for the convicted killer of a doctor in the US. No
action has been taken against them by the hierarchy.

Where, you wonder, is the Vatican's "pro-life" condemnation
of criminal attacks on clinics and their staff, including murder,
or those who seek to justify or cover up these attacks? If the
hierarchy are not directly responsible for the propaganda,
violence and intimidation, why do they not issue guidelines for
appropriate behaviour by protesters outside clinics? Where is the
acknowledgement of the suffering and deaths of so many women
who are forced to carry a pregnancy that will not produce a
healthy baby, or where they cannot deliver safely? How do they
weigh up the losses from so many desperate illegal abortions, the
result of their bans on contraception? Where is the understanding
that many children are born only to suffer and die because of this?
And where is the care for the women, the attempt to understand
their need, or support for those who help them? To an outsider,
as for many good Catholics, it makes no sense at all: plenty of
removing mountains but strictly no charity.

Some have argued that this is all a reaction to what Church
members are actually doing. The less their members obey their
dogmas, the more the authorities are determined to use their
political influence to block contraception and abortion for
members and non-members alike. The hierarchy is unrelenting.
Under the banner of Life, this is a fight to the death.

Change is coming – for gays but not for women

A flurry of excitement greeted moves by Pope Francis, at his inauguration, to re-emphasise the need to listen to the poor. However, although he is less judgmental about individual "sins" he shows little or no understanding of the lives of poor women, or the decisions they face throughout their lives. Observers within the Church have concluded that he is personally opposed to any freedom of action on contraception. Indeed, he recently called on married couples to "be fruitful and multiply", and not spend time looking after cats and dogs when they could be having children. He also claimed that if a couple remained childless they would ultimately have nothing but "the bitterness of loneliness". It is a surprising threat, coming from a man who is a lifelong celibate with no family and certainly no children. Is the celibate life then so unbearable?

A Vatican survey issued in November 2013, under Pope Francis, asked how people were receiving the Church's messages on family matters, ahead of a Family Synod in 2014, which would put particular emphasis on homosexuality and sexual relationships outside marriage. The question on contraception, though, was: "How can a more open attitude towards having children be fostered? How can an increase in births be promoted?" Again it is the focus on numbers and not individuals, with no reference to the health of the mother or the welfare of the children and families. If even more births are the answer, what is the question? Perhaps it is "How can we force women to have more children than is good for them or for their families?"

So although the hierarchy can change, or at least think about changing, its attitude to gay people and relationships, or the abuse of children by priests – or even appointing a few women to positions in the Church – it shows no sign of rethinking its commitment to maximising births. Perhaps the most one can expect from the current Catholic hierarchy is to reduce the vast amounts of Church funds which go into the campaigns against international or national programmes for women's choice.

They could issue a call to "pro-lifers" to stop harassing women, threatening the clinics or justifying arson and murder, and pushing a distorted version of pregnancy and birth. For the rest, it would require Francis and the bishops to do a different kind of "listening to the poor" which would mean listening to poor women in order to understand who they are, how they live, and why they make the decisions they do. One recent statement by Pope Francis allowed priests to forgive women for abortions. However, the language used was that of right wing abortion opponents in the United States: "The tragedy of abortion is experienced by some with a superficial awareness, as if not realizing the extreme harm that such an act entails. Many others, on the other hand, although experiencing this moment as a defeat, believe that they have no other option. I think in particular of all the women who have resorted to abortion." This is the assumption that women are "victims" because they cannot make informed decisions about their own lives. It perhaps speaks loudly of the lobbying to which Francis is subjected on the matter by conservative men rather than an ability to listen to the millions of women who make their own choices.

Those liberal Catholic commentators who hope for a more substantive relaxation of the official position on this, emphasise the role in Church teachings of the *"sensus fidelium"*, the common sense of the faithful Church members based on their own experience and conscience. (The Spanish have a saying: "An ounce of mother is worth more than a pound of clergy.") They cite the example of how this can work in the case of the centuries-old ban on the "sin of usury" – charging interest on loans. This teaching was quietly dropped as Church members persisted in borrowing and lending with interest. In fact the Church now has its own bank, which commits usury all day, every day. So much for a supposed sin, conveniently forgotten when the notion becomes ridiculous. Or as an English saying has it: if you can't beat them, join them.

Gudorf comments that with most Church members using contraception if they can, and abortion when necessary, in the future the hierarchy could come to recognise that their members are right and that the biosphere is threatened by the sheer number of its teeming human inhabitants. They could, she suggests, "discern the will of God and the presence of the Spirit" in the choices of those who "share responsibility for the lives and health and prosperity of future generations" by having few children, or none.

It is interesting that many Catholic nuns understand the issues far better than the hierarchy. Nuns in the US, who work mainly with the most disadvantaged women and men, have united to issue a statement justifying contraception. There are reports of subversion among nuns in Catholic hospitals: a friend told me she knew someone in hospital in Germany, for treatment after a botched abortion, who was talking to a nun in the next bed. The nun whispered to her: "Why don't you use the 'Mary Magdalen' technique? All the prostitutes use it." This was cotton wool coated with oil. It is perhaps not the most sophisticated method, and quite old-fashioned, but most certainly better than nothing.

Others are much more pessimistic about any real change at the top. Catholics for Choice observes: "The Catholic hierarchy has its own politics. In a world where power is sought after and ordained for the long term, taking a reactionary stance on controversial issues can be rewarding – the old guard gets to preserve the status quo, while newcomers rise faster when not making waves. On a deeper level, however, the all-male, celibate hierarchy can avoid any honest confrontation about sexuality by insisting that sex is simply a function of procreation."

The hierarchy is still deaf to the needs of the people. I am reminded of the Bible's saying from Jesus: "If a son shall ask bread of any of you that is a father, will he give him a stone?" (*Matthew*, 7:9) In an open letter of 2008, fifty pro-choice Catholic organisations in different countries wrote that the ban on contraception "has had catastrophic effects on the poor and weak of the whole world, putting in danger the lives of women and exposing millions of people to the risk of contracting HIV." There has been no response from Rome.

Frances Kissling, President of Catholics for a Free Choice, was asked whether the Church had been mostly a force for good or a force for ill. She replied: "There are certainly days when I believe that the institution is so deeply corrupted that it should be destroyed. I think of all the ways in which people who have been part of this Church have been abused: priests who want to get married, women who want to be priests, women who use contraception, gay people. At the same time, some of the very same people who can be so abusive to their family have done great social good: Catholic education, Catholic health care. There are parts of the world where the only place you will be medically treated is by a Catholic. It does enormous good and enormous evil."

Resources

Professor Daniel C Maguire, "The Moderate Roman Catholic Position on Contraception and Abortion" Marquette University (available on the internet).

Frederic Ballenegger, "The Ethics and Theology of Population Dynamics," unpublished paper, 12 December 2012.

Christine Gudorf, *Body, Sex and Pleasure: Reconstructing Christian Sexual Ethics* (Pilgrim Press, 1995).

 "Letter to the Bishops of the Catholic Church on the Collaboration of Men and Women in the Church and in the World", 2004, signed by Cardinal Joseph Ratzinger [now the retired Pope Benedict XVI] and Angelo Amato, and approved by Pope John Paul II.

Andrew Brown, "The War against Pope Francis," *The Guardian*, London, 28 October 2017.

Stephen D Mumford, "The Life and Death of NSSM 200: How the Destruction of Political Will Doomed a US Population Policy," (Amazon.com, 1996).

PART THREE: THE BATTLES

Chapter six

THE GLOBAL GAG
"Pro-life" Adamants impose silence

Everyone – especially every woman – needs to be able to decide whether to have children, and when would be the best time. It is essential for our own health and welfare, for good sexual and family relationships, and to support ourselves, our families and our communities. It underpins equal rights in society and the workplace, freeing women from unwanted pregnancies and the struggle to maintain the resulting children. Modern contraception is also essential to stabilise our population numbers. It is not so long ago that Europe was exporting large numbers of its people to colonies all around the world, with all the enduring conflict that still continues from that process. Now it is the poorest countries that have the highest rates of human population growth. Stabilising our numbers is essential if we are to preserve our whole environment, not just for our own benefit but as a legacy to future generations.

So why – when richer women can now have contraception and poorer women do not – is there such a guilty silence in the media and in international circles about the issue? Some of the organisations which should be discussing it have made it a taboo subject. This is in spite of the fact that there have been massive advances in the contraceptive methods available, and improvements in service delivery to meet people's needs effectively and safely, in even the poorest areas of the world. But this information is regarded as something not for discussion in polite society – an old-fashioned approach to sex and contraception that seems bizarre in our highly sexualised, porn-filled world. The knowledge of these advances seems to be confined to those working directly in sexual health services and is being ignored by many women's and environmental groups – and by too many governments and international agencies that are supposedly working to eradicate poverty.

All too often we hear the defensive line about this being to do with supposed "population control". In fact nobody on the international scene is advocating this – it is a thing of the past. The single exception is the Chinese Government and its forced "one child" policy, and even this has now finally been relaxed to two children. We can hardly blame the family planning movement for the policies of the Chinese Government. The real reason for the international reluctance to discuss the issues, I suggest, is an enormous inhibition or avoidance created by the obsessions, and sometimes the sheer aggression, of the "pro-lifers". These are made up of individuals, organisations, right wing governments and some major religious forces like the Catholic Church and, increasingly, other fundamentalist Christian, Muslim and other groups. They are the real controlling force in this debate, they have enormous amounts of money and they are highly organised.

Like all reactionary movements, it starts with propaganda: untruths endlessly repeated, together with the repetitive use of language that hides the reality. With the opposition to contraception and abortion it starts with endless repetition of myths about "unborn babies", "unborn children" or the "preborn". This is a denial of the crucial importance of birth as the start of a life, and a contradiction to how all human societies view the start of a baby's life, in law and in the real world. It is birth that transforms a foetus into a baby. An "unborn baby" is a contradiction in terms.

All human cultures celebrate birth. They aim to support the health and wellbeing of women who are pregnant so that at the end they can finally give birth to a child that will survive into adulthood. Our lives as humans start with our birth: this is the common-sense view, and always has been. People worldwide have always celebrated the birth of a baby as a momentous event: a new member of a family, community and society: a tiny new human being that we can see, touch and celebrate. A child can be part of the family and community only once she or he is born.

The opposition work hard to give the impression that a fully-formed baby is in the womb almost from the moment of conception and is merely "growing" in preparation for birth. Pope Francis, among many others, has spoken of "an innocent child growing in the mother's womb". They use cleverly angled pictures of foetuses, blown up to the size of a fully developed baby and not the tiny embryo or undeveloped foetus it really is, to give that impression. For these ideologues, birth is irrelevant and makes no real difference to the "preborn" or "unborn baby". Therefore, they argue, even from the moment of conception the supposed "unborn baby" or "the preborn" is a fully developed human being. They argue that its rights are therefore the same as, or even greater than the people who are already living their own independent lives – especially the mother carrying the foetus, and giving it life as part of her own body. Their case is based on a kind of propaganda that falsifies pictures, distorts language and is highly selective and dishonest in its use of scans and other modern medical techniques.

We now know that at conception, where the sperm fertilises the egg, it becomes a single-celled organism called a zygote. Over the next two weeks there is a germinal period, during which the cell divides into two to create a multi-celled organism called a blastocyst that then moves down the fallopian tube and has to implant into the woman's womb in order to develop further. This may develop to form one individual, or two identical twins (and occasionally triplets). Implantation occurs when the cells nestle into the uterine lining and rupture tiny blood vessels. The connective web of blood vessels and membranes that form between them will provide nourishment for the developing being for the next nine months. If the process goes well (and there are many failures of implantation) the next stage is a tiny unformed embryo, which then finally develops into a foetus. This gradually develops the nervous system and brain, sex organs, vital organs like liver, kidneys and heart, and the physical shape that will be necessary for independent life. At the end of the whole nine-month process, once the foetus has grown large enough and the lungs are finally developed, it will be ready to be born as a baby.

Until the mother gives birth to the foetus she has been carrying, whether conventionally or through surgery, it is on life support from her. This means it is entirely dependent on her existence, her breathing, her nutrition, her internal organs, her blood, and her health and wellbeing. If she thrives, the foetus has the best possible chance of thriving also. If she starves, the foetus starves. If she dies (unless it can be rescued by a caesarean birth) it will die with her. In a very real sense, the unborn foetus belongs to the mother since its body is a part of hers.

Modern medical research and practice has shown what a momentous event the birth of a baby actually is. At birth newborns become independent human beings, living and breathing on their own. They are expelled from the birth canal with liquid in their lungs: the sudden change of temperature and environment triggers a reaction in the central nervous system which prompts them to take their first breath within about ten seconds after birth.

This expands their lungs and dramatically lowers the blood pressure in parts of their heart and other organs, switching their intake of oxygen and changing the circulation of blood – a process which takes about three minutes. They will then have an entirely new cardiovascular system, which will be the basis of their whole life. Their nutrition will no longer be derived from their mother's through the placenta, but must be obtained independently whether from the mother's milk or other foods. All their organs, especially the liver, heart and lungs, must now start operating independently, or not at all.

Through modern medical procedures of life support involving the latest (and most expensive) technology, we have been able to push back the date at which a baby can be born prematurely, without fully developed organs, but still survive. We may have reached the limits of what is possible for premature births: it is considered unlikely that we can reduce these techniques to even lower ages of gestation.

Even the Catholic Church, now so vehement about "unborn babies", has always dated a child's life from the moment of their birth and refused, until very recently, to allow baptism for miscarried foetuses or babies who die during the birth. For centuries, when child mortality was extremely high, the churches even used to delay baptism of a baby until it was certain that she or he would survive the first few days and be able to live into the future.

That basic logic about the start of life is now being challenged by the "pro-lifers" with a very ancient idea, arising from ignorance of human reproduction, that women were merely containers or "vessels" for a man's sperm, contributing nothing of their own to the future baby. There are strong overtones of the "vessel" image in much of what the Catholic Church and many fundamentalists are saying on this subject now: that the "unborn" are more important than the women who carry and nurture them, and give them life.

As vessels or containers, women can be treated almost as equipment for the production of babies, and even as appendages to the "unborn" – without dignity and without choice. Even if a woman's health, or even her life, is threatened by the pregnancy, she must be forced to continue it. If she is married but not pregnant, she should be "encouraged" to join the club. Hence the increasingly adamant Catholic ban on modern contraception, and its ferocious opposition to termination once pregnancy is even suspected. It sometimes appears as if the men in the hierarchy are seeing any children as "ours", to be protected at all costs, unlike the women who are "other" and of less importance. It enables a focus on numbers and not on nurture.

This is the subject of vicious battles in the US, which are reaching levels of absurdity and where, in November 2017, Republicans in the House of Representatives passed extremist foetal "personhood" language as part of a tax bill. The US Senate considered a separate plan that similarly considers an "unborn child...at any stage of development" (from the moment of conception as a fertilised egg) as a tax beneficiary, in a move that takes the campaign against women's reproductive rights to the level of wanting to give them National Insurance numbers. Is this a new version of the Invasion of the Body-snatchers?

This was certainly the view of the Romanian dictator Nicolae Ceausescu, who imposed the investigation of any miscarriages, criminalised abortion and contraception, and subjected girls and women to monthly gynaecological examinations to identify and monitor pregnancies. "The foetus is the socialist property of the whole society," he declared. "Giving birth is a patriotic duty ... Those who refuse to have children are deserters." The result was the highest rate of maternal deaths in Europe, huge numbers of orphans and abandoned children whose families could not care for them, and a wave of dangerous abortions.

The old, pre-scientific notion of women as containers for independent "unborn children" has become a staple of right wing masculinist movements, which are often fiercely opposed to women's equality and independence. Racist ideas of eugenics – increasing "our" numbers in a battle with "the other" – are often raised by fascist movements. In Italy, for example, right wing skinheads are reported to have attended a rally where they used the fascist salute of one outstretched arm, some of them wearing a "9%" badge – a classic eugenic reference to the percentage of the world population that is "white". A climate of aggression and fear in Italy is having an effect on medical services: seven out of ten doctors there now say they would refuse to carry out terminations of pregnancy, whatever the risks of that pregnancy or the needs of the woman concerned. The refusals have been rising, from 59% in 2005 to 70% in 2013, and have led to a predictable increase in the number of desperate women self-administering or having illegal abortions. One woman who was admitted to an Italian hospital for termination of a pregnancy, where the foetus had no chance of surviving beyond birth, was forced to wait for several days in induced labour for the one doctor who would help her to come on shift.

Since there has been no rise in religious affiliation in Italy (quite the opposite) and no indication that doctors are becoming more religious, it appears that the doctors are increasingly worried about their career prospects and even their safety in the face of increasingly aggressive Antis.

The "unborn" and the United States

The battle over control of women and the "unborn" is going on in almost every part of the world. However, the country where this fight has become most bitter is the United States, where right wing Christian fundamentalists and evangelicals have joined the Catholic bishops in their campaign. Michelle Goldberg has suggested that this move represented a fierce backlash against rapid social change in general, and the women's movement in particular: "As a synecdoche for American social chaos, abortion was a powerful political motivator."

Although contraception and abortion are legal in the US, clinics which provide these services find themselves under sustained misrepresentation and attack. Death threats from the "pro-lifers" are daily occurrences. Some of the more violent activists have carried out murders of doctors and clinic staff, by means of arson, bombs and shooting – using the tactics of terrorism. Between 1977 and mid 2016 there were 11 killings, 26 attempted murders, 42 bombings, 185 cases of arson, and thousands more incidents of criminal behaviour including threats, smears, harassment and intimidation. They include publicising the personal details and addresses of clinic staff and even information on their children.

The attacks have been escalating, especially after the release of propaganda videos in 2015, deliberately falsified to claim that clinics "murder children" and sell "baby parts". A security firm identified more than 25,000 incidents of online threats to clinics and staff in just six weeks. One anonymous caller to a hospital switchboard said: "We will kill all abortion doctors." Another threatened to set all the clinics on fire. The threats are realistic, since all this has indeed happened; they inspire great fear and have indeed driven many doctors and health staff out of the work. One family planning doctor found her name, personal and professional details and photos of herself and her child on an anti-choice website, which claimed she was part of an "abortion cartel". "There is no better way to intimidate and incite fear than to target a family member, especially a child. The message is unambiguous: I'm being watched, and so is my daughter."

Intimidation extends also to the media. A children's author, Judy Blume, who has spoken out in defence of the Planned Parenthood organisation, had over 700 hate-mail warnings: "We know where you are going to be and we'll be there waiting for you." Planned Parenthood's Fred Clarkson researched the anti-abortion militias in the United States and was invited onto a major TV network to speak about it. This was cancelled at short notice "because they'd have angry pro-life viewers calling in and they didn't want to take that heat".

The FBI and local police have been involved in trying to stop all this, and have been involved in protecting clinics and breaking up groups of people who were blockading the entrances, but so far have had little control of the situation. Attempts to prosecute the people creating the worst video have come to nothing. Many family planning services have been forced to spend a fortune on security or even to close down clinics altogether, especially those in the poorest areas of the country and those serving the women of black and minority groups, who have the least chance of travelling somewhere else for help.

The battles are also raging in State legislatures, and in the courts. The pro-choice side are constantly being forced to fight to preserve what they have. One landmark decision in June 2016 saw the US Supreme Court striking down extreme restrictions on access to abortion by the State of Texas – but there will be many more such attempts, and with the appointment of conservative judges by President Trump the decisions are more likely to go the other way in future. For women in the United States this is a difficult time, having to fight again to safeguard what they have previously fought for and won.

Troy Newman of Operation Rescue has spoken excitedly about the successes he and his allies have made in restricting access to abortion across the country. "We got Trump elected — we put a lot of effort into that, we're putting Supreme Court justices in place, and now stacking legislation that is going to end abortion as we know it," he said. "I think these guys should be very worried they'll soon end up in jail."

At the same time, the anti-choice crusade is being exported from the US as many conservative evangelical Christians expand their reach – especially in Latin America – with many of them campaigning hard against abortion in particular and family planning services in general. They have the money, they have the people and they have the conviction of their own righteousness, which for some means anything is permitted, up to and including murder.

The war over women and foetuses in the US has now reached the government itself, with US President Donald Trump saying during his campaign that abortion ought to be illegal and that women who undergo such a procedure should face "some sort of punishment". Faced with a barrage of criticism, he then retreated by saying that the doctors and health staff should be held criminally responsible. His Vice-President, Mike Pence, and key political appointments including Ambassador to the United Nations and Secretary of Health, have a track record of opposition to contraception and all forms of pregnancy termination.

During his campaign, Trump created a Catholic advisory group filled with some of the most vehement anti-choice advocates in the US. It included John Klink who, during his time as advisor to the Holy See Mission to the United Nations, used his position of influence to ensure that "the wave of so-called 'reproductive and sexual rights' would [not] be enshrined as new 'fundamental' human rights," and Austin Ruse, who stated with regard to anti-abortion issues, "Trump will let our side do exactly what we want to do." He was referring mainly to domestic provision for women, but indeed Trump has acted quickly on the international scene, "projecting ideology onto global health programs," as Brian Dixon of the Population Connection Action Fund has described it. The result, he predicted, would be the closure of clinics in huge areas of the developing world, with a shortage of medication, increases in diseases like AIDS, malaria and TB, and needless suffering. Failure to provide good contraception would also lead to increases in abortion, almost all of it in dangerous circumstances that would cost many women's lives.

President Trump's "Global Gag Rule" (officially named "Protecting Life in Global Health Assistance") requires any non-governmental organisations that receive US funds to stop providing, referring to, or even sharing information about abortion, even if it is legal in that country and paid from non-US funds. So much for freedom of expression and the Second Amendment to the US Constitution. This is an even more extreme version of a policy first introduced under President Reagan, which had led to the closure of many health services providing basic health and maternity care, often in the poorest and most inaccessible areas. The gag had been removed by President Obama. Since the US is the largest source of humanitarian aid worldwide, and especially since it seeks to silence those funded by other donors, the Global Gag policy sets back health provision across the globe, and especially any help with modern contraception. Alongside the gag rule, the US Administration is proposing to cut over $600 million in direct funding for family planning, and scrap the financial contribution to the UN Population Fund (UNFPA).

The good news for women is that there is strong opposition in the US Congress to Trump's actions, and future Administrations are likely to soften or repeal them. Meanwhile, other aid donor countries moved quickly to replace the lost funds from the US Government, although this merely seeks to rescue existing programmes when there was already a desperate need for expansion. Thank you Sweden, Denmark, Finland, Netherlands, Belgium, Luxembourg, Canada and Cape Verde. But much more support is needed, not just to make up the US funding cuts but to safeguard the non-governmental work and to extend the programmes to all areas, if women's and families' needs for health and family planning are to be met.

So where are the women?

Faced with this barrage of propaganda and extremism it is very sad, though perhaps not really surprising, that so many women's organisations have turned their backs on the issues of pregnancy and birth, and how we can control the fertility that nature has given us. In the case of Germaine Greer, in what is perhaps her most ill-informed book *Sex and Destiny*, she idealises poor families with many children, misunderstands the contraceptive methods available, argues that the women should not use any form of birth control, and seriously suggests that abstaining from sex would be the answer anyway. The last idea is a staple of conservative approaches to the issue.

In most of the richer countries the battles for family planning have been won, and most women can take for granted that we can have sex without getting pregnant, with the option of the "morning-after" pill or termination at an early stage if contraception fails. Our whole life is managed on the basis that we do not have to be pregnant if we do not want to, and can therefore have as much control over our own lives as men do. However, this security means that we seem to have forgotten what it was like without that. We either ignore the problems of women who do not have it, or in the case of Germaine Greer and a few others they even argue for double standards: contraception for us but not for them.

While countless column inches and many hours of broadcast time in rich countries are devoted to promoting fertility among women who cannot conceive when they want to, and big money is invested in IVF (in-vitro fertilisation) and fertility research, contraception gets almost no media attention and far too little money. Where there have been political battles for women's reproductive rights in the West, they have been around abortion. Some abortion activists in the West say they do not need to talk about contraception because the debate on that is over. The problem is: for poorer women, especially in the poorer countries, it has hardly begun.

So what about the internationally based non-governmental organisations? Surely they will be advocating the best possible contraception for all? Unfortunately, this is really where the problem lies. Many of them are avoiding the issues, thus offering a perfect excuse for the rest of the international development community to do the same. They have failed to understand what modern programmes and methods are really offering women. Some aid organisations have stopped providing any form of family planning, even when they have done it in the past. Looking just at the UK-based agencies, for example, even though the UK Government is at the forefront of funding family planning worldwide, confusion reigns. Oxfam UK, which used to offer contraception services, has now retreated:"We leave it to others," according to a representative I contacted. The problem is, in many of the areas where they work, there are no others (or at best the tender mercies of a Catholic clinic or hospital). The Catholic aid agency CAFOD predictably offers no help to women. Womankind organises support groups for women in several different countries, but no access to family planning services at all. Save the Children provides contraception, but not abortion. Meanwhile, however, Christian Aid – which itself faces strong negative pressures from some of the churches which support it – courageously asserts:"We believe that reproductive healthcare should be provided in the context of high-quality primary healthcare for women, men and their children." So there is no consistency, and for many areas where there are British voluntary aid programmes, any help with planning for children is specifically excluded.

The women's international lobby sends representatives to UN meetings to successfully push issues like female genital mutilation (FGM), rape, domestic violence, or women's rights at work, both nationally and internationally. They are often funded and supported by their own governments. Many of them, sadly, have nothing to say about women's rights to decide when to get pregnant, and will try to block any attempts to raise the issue. I wrote a piece (at their request) about poor women's need for good contraception, for the co-ordinating group, The Association for Women's Rights in Development (AWID). Disappointingly – but not surprisingly – it never appeared and their silence on this issue continues. AWID describes itself as "the only international feminist organisation in the world" with member organisations in 163 countries. Maintaining international silence about one of the key issues for women seems to be what they are really about. In this respect they are lined up with Trump and his Global Gag.

No surprises there, because it is the established pattern with many national and international women's organisations. Often it will be a few individuals within the group who react violently against any discussion of contraception. A small group of US-based "radical" women, the Women's Environment and Development Organisation, caused problems at the 1992 Earth Summit with their adamant opposition to any mention of population growth or women's right to contraception, which they managed to block. The strength of opposition among the few means that the majority will back off, and it becomes a subject to be avoided. Since there is such a taboo against discussing the issues, many of the organisations still seem to believe that we are living in a past where indeed there were attempts by the US in particular at "population control" – an approach which has long been abandoned as counter-productive.

Some in these organisations have opposed family planning across the board because contraceptive trials were allegedly conducted with African women. There is a true double standard here since they are not suggesting that western women should boycott contraception for that reason. There is also a notion that contraception is dangerous to a woman who is malnourished. I had one conversation with a leading international feminist where she came out with this last one. I pointed out that the most dangerous thing for this woman would actually be pregnancy, especially if it was unwanted. This seemed to be a completely new idea for her – to her credit, she was open to reviewing her whole approach to the issue. If only all the women involved would do the same.

This is largely about wilful avoidance of this topic. However, if we try to understand why this is happening, we have to acknowledge the huge range of issues the women's organisations are facing in advancing and defending women's rights, while trying to make women central to development. Their attention is increasingly being focused on the horrors of war for women – especially the murder, rape, kidnap and enslavement of women, which is increasingly a part of modern warfare. The horrible conditions for many women and their children who are refugees from war is another cause for concern. Then there are the single-issue campaigns like female genital mutilation (FGM), sexual exploitation, domestic violence or forced marriage, which are seen to have a better chance of success than tackling all the issues at once. Defending the rights of lesbians and transsexuals has also become important, as have the rights of sex workers. Community activism, the environment and opposition to harmful development, especially for indigenous people, is a particular focus for some women's groups. All of these are important issues, although not a justification for ignoring one of the most critical ones.

Women's rights advocates in some developing countries are also facing a right wing authoritarian backlash aimed at reversing hard-won women's rights. There have been murders and death threats to women who are human rights defenders. These have caused great concern throughout the movement, which feels an urgent need to support and defend these activists. Much effort has had to be spent on defending the advances already made and, for many groups in Third World countries, the challenge is merely to survive in a hostile environment.

This is also about money. All the international women's organisations are financially weak, and all too conscious that their budgets are a fraction of the money available to the big development agencies and the environmental organisations. There has been an overall decrease in funding to women's organisations from official bilateral and multilateral aid agencies arising from the 2008 global financial crisis, the increasing numbers of conservative governments, and public pressure in the rich countries to reduce foreign aid for developing countries. At the same time the efforts of many have shifted from campaigning on global issues to working in particular areas on practical projects, as women and girls become recognised as central to the global development agenda. Economic issues predominate: land rights, legal issues, access to education, finance, markets and working conditions. All of these are important, but the fact that none of this will work if women cannot control the number and timing of their children has not been sufficiently understood.

The reality is that many women in the international voluntary organisations are tired, distracted and overwhelmed. The energy needed for a rethink on reproductive issues is just not there for some of the most hard-pressed. Some of them, especially in the richer countries, have lost their open-mindedness and their campaigning edge as their organisations become more professionalised. They were originally set up and run mainly by committed volunteers who could say what they liked, but now there are paid staff, often young and insecure, occupying jobs in international development for which there is fierce competition.

They have money to earn, rent to pay, their own children to support, careers to nurture. Are they going to rock the boat? If there is even one colleague who objects? Or if they go to a conference and face a fierce attack by a Third World individual or organisation accusing them of wanting "population control"? The answer too often is: no way.

Such debates can become vicious and intensely personal. There are a few organisations with close ties to the "pro-lifers" and with the money to attend all the international conferences. One such organisation loudly proclaims projects such as "the Virtual Mural for Abortion Rights!" (everything comes with a distancing!) but also "attacks the population control mentality and the development of contraceptive vaccines from a feminist point of view". It is doubtful whether women facing unmanageable pregnancies would agree that this is a pro-women or feminist point of view.

The women's movement (like other movements for social change) has always had bitter disputes, and if you experience even one of these you tend to avoid other potential confrontations. It is all too easy for the Antis to put women off even mentioning fertility issues, let alone having a proper discussion. And so it is that much of the international women's movement – which should be leading the campaign for family planning worldwide – maintains silence.

The population people

There are, of course, important exceptions to the avoidance of family planning issues. Many women's organisations in poor countries, notably in Latin America and the Caribbean, have been vociferous in their demands for contraception and a general opening up of health services to the poorest women.

There are voluntary family planning associations working tirelessly in almost every country in the world to introduce clinic services and to lobby their own local authorities and governments to fund these on a bigger scale. They are backed by a network of international support organisations, which include their own International Planned Parent Federation (IPPF) and the United Nations Fund for Population (UNFPA) together with many national and international organisations specifically working to improve women's access to services. They have been joined by some big donors, including the Gates Foundation, which handles some of Microsoft founder Bill Gates's millions. They are supporting family planning programmes in some of the poorest countries that have the least support, and financing research and lobbying work. All of these are campaigning for understanding and support on contraception and sexual health under the Sexual and Reproductive Health and Rights (SRHR) banner as an integral element in international development.

These organisations do brilliant work, developing contraception delivery and outreach while monitoring outcomes and researching the needs and the issues. In 2015 they finally managed, after many years of trying and failing, to get reproductive health as one of the UN's Sustainable Development Goals (SDGs) for international development, with the target by 2030 to "ensure universal access to sexual and reproductive health-care services, including for family planning, information and education, and the integration of reproductive health into national strategies and programmes." It was a great leap forward, but constant work is needed to make sure it is implemented against relentless opposition.

These organisations are not communicating enough with development economists and practitioners, the international health and "One Health" sector, or environmentalists. The population people (and their organisations often use the word "population" in their names) talk mainly to each other. They campaign with, and speak to, mainly other specialist groups in their own field. My immersion in their social media conversations reveals a morass of jargon and initials which are never explained, and which no outsider would know. This unfortunately includes the terms "reproductive health" or "SRHR" which are not well understood in general development circles or the wider world.

The family planning organisations have generally failed to engage with women's organisations, even to the extent of informing them of what is happening in their field. They collectively give the impression of staying in their comfort zone, preaching to the converted and staying well away from the nasty opposition. The conspiracy of silence about what is really happening in the field is feeding the taboos against discussion. Martha Campbell, who has been centrally involved in all of this, has described the current situation as "a perfect storm of silence" adopted by family planning organisations as a way to preserve services, but which in reality has lost them vital support. She points to the run-up to the 1994 Cairo conference (UN International Conference on Population and Development, or ICPD). "Talking about population became politically incorrect in many circles. Drawing attention to any connection between population growth and environmental destruction became taboo…"

This taboo is blocking what could be life-saving work. There seems to be little awareness among many women's organisations of the hugely beneficial impact that women's groups on the ground can have if they work together for family planning and sexual health. As the organisation Women and Children First concludes, women's groups working on these issues in poor areas can transform lives: "Where at least 30% of pregnant women took part in the groups, maternal deaths can be reduced by up to 49% and newborn deaths by a third." With such dramatic improvements in lives saved, it is ironic that women in so many national and international organisations – who themselves would not dream of giving up their own choices about sexuality and whether to have children – are turning their backs on the issue just when their support is most needed to give all women that choice. Double standards for rich and poor women are all too prevalent, and simply not acceptable.

At a time when the family planning community is under extreme pressure over funding, especially in the United States, it is crucial that they break the silence.

Environmentalists, where are you?

In the 1960s and 1970s several environmental writers warned of the "population explosion" or "Population Bomb" as described in Paul and Anne Ehrlich's influential book of that name published in 1968. The problem of how to feed, house and employ rapidly increasing numbers of people, while preserving natural resources and habitats in the face of rapid climate change and global conflicts, is indeed critical to all people and the whole environment. Yet many environmental organisations and commentators have now turned their backs on the issue, deciding, according to the veteran campaigner Dave Foreman, that "overpopulation worry is kicked into the corner and shunned like an old, smelly dog." What happened?

I can only conclude that – like the women's organisations – many environmentalists have backed away from unpleasant confrontations. Take the near-civil war within the Sierra Club in the United States. Previously strongly supportive of work to help people stabilise their family size, its Board was infiltrated in the 1990s by white supremacists with overtly racist views who wanted to turn this into an anti-immigration campaign. "When you talk about population," said Larry Fahn, Sierra Club president during some of the bitterest infighting, "the immigration people come out of the woodwork with their hate mongering. It's unfortunate that the subject brings out a racist agenda." The outcome was a virtual prohibition on discussion of human population increase and its impact on the environment. A more effective approach would have been to tackle the question of people's decisions about children on its own, and not link it to the immigration into the richer countries. It is a mistake that several groups have made in the past and it is an unnecessary distraction.

Since the link between human numbers and the natural environment is obvious, environmentalists have had to look hard for excuses for their avoidance. Some of these go beyond even what the women's groups are saying. The "deep green" writer George Monbiot, while claiming that western over-consumption is the only cause of environmental destruction and climate change, has even written that highlighting women's rights, the need for family planning and the expanding human population means "blaming the victims". This is taking self-justification to absurd lengths. We will not be silenced by you, George.

These (mainly male) environmentalists do have one obvious get-out clause, of course: that the international women's movement has failed to raise the issues effectively. Some of the men have even described the women as "pro-natalist" which is certainly an exaggeration: apart from Germaine Greer the women's groups are not advocating more births, they are avoiding the issue altogether. It is far too easy (and dishonest) for the environmental movement, which is enormously big, professional, well financed and powerful, to blame the struggling women's organisations for their own inadequacies.

It is very unfortunate that the key book on this topic, Anne and Paul Ehrlichs' "Population Bomb," has in the end proved counter-productive in trying to get environmentalists to focus on the issue. The book predicted worldwide famine in the 1970s, which would kill hundreds of millions of people. Predictions are always risky and this one did not happen – or at least not on the scale they suggested. Even more serious than this was their advocacy of the now abandoned policy of "population control", including forcing Indian fathers of three or more children to be sterilised. This has allowed many to dismiss their, and other people's, warnings about human population increases, and to ridicule any notion that large numbers of people could ever run out of food.

Some claim that technological advances will be developed to allow ever-increasing numbers of people to be fed. Many argue that environmental destruction is purely a problem of over-consumption by rich consumers, despite some very persuasive analysis by colleagues showing that the increasing numbers of very poor people are also a major factor. Indeed, the desperation of people without land, employment or place in society is driving them to take over and degrade huge areas of land previously left to wildlife and nature, such as rainforests and semi-deserts – precisely the areas that environmentalists are so worried about.

Another favoured argument, especially among the men, is that synthetic oestrogens in some hormonal contraceptives are getting into the rivers via sewage treatment plants, and may be interfering with the reproduction of some fish. I am waiting for these men to campaign for the obvious alternative of barrier methods that do not use hormones, including condoms and male sterilisation. Most of them would not even be using barrier methods themselves. Instead: leave it to the women, and then blame them!

There is probably some truth in the claim about oestrogen, although the widely used chemical Bisphenol A is also suspected of having this effect on fish. The definitive environmental answer to the anti-hormone argument has been humorously but clearly set out by Umbra Fisk in the online environmental magazine Grist. She argues that effective contraception is so vital to individuals and the planet that it offsets even some environmental damage. "Preventing the creation of another resource-using, carbon-emitting human is by far the eco-friendliest step anyone can take, even if you create a tower of condom wrappers to do so... Just go forth and don't be fruitful." She discusses different methods in some detail, balancing effectiveness as well as environmental effects, and recommends the latest intrauterine devices (IUDs) while "still, given how well it works, the Pill and its ilk remain a viable option". Is this controversial stuff? No, it is environmental common sense.

The avoidance of human population issues by so many in the environmental movement has been described by Professor Roger Martin as "telling a silent lie every time they put out a statement on some environmental problem where they know that every additional person makes it harder and ultimately impossible to solve." As with the women's organisations, he finds a partial explanation in the increasing professionalisation of the field. As the previous head of an environmental organisation himself: "When I started with a staff of three, I was a hard-hitting campaigner with a lot of volunteers. By the time I finished ten years later with a staff of 35, my priority concern, if I'm honest, had switched from preserving the wildlife of Somerset to keeping my staff and myself in work. So not upsetting funders became more and more important, and it made us ever more toothless watchdogs. And I think that's happened to the Sierra Club and many others. They've become part of the Establishment, they don't rock boats." The desperation to hold on to funding by avoiding anything controversial is also emphasised by Ed Barry of the US Population Institute: "Many conservation and nongovernmental organizations that run on member support, even the big ones, shy away from the population issue. That's because it puts their funding at risk." Sadly, the scramble for funding has overwhelmed their integrity.

The fact that the environmental movement is very male-dominated means they are embarrassed about discussing women, especially women's bodies, sexuality and birth. In documentaries about nature they are very happy to show pictures of animals mating, but cannot bring themselves to discuss sex and reproduction among humans. Jonathan Porritt, another leading environmentalist, has admitted: "Population raises all these questions about religion, about culture, about male dominance in the world; and [we] get very uncomfortable about that."

George Monbiot has also admitted that human population is "an important issue most Greens will not discuss. Is this sensitivity or is it cowardice? Perhaps a bit of both." And so the great avoidance of this issue becomes ever more entrenched – even though many of those involved are not even quite sure why, and perhaps are afraid to ask. The old accusing slogans of "eugenics" and "population control" are put out there, a bit like waving garlic and a cross in front of the witches, zombies and vampires in horror movies.

These words help to build convenient "straw men":

pretending that promoting choice is somehow evil and so worthy of contempt and attack. Setting up a "straw man" in an argument is pretending the other side is saying something it is not, constructing a weak position that you claim they hold and then proceeding to demolish it. It is deeply dishonest, and it is embedded in the anti-choice position. Take, for example, a statement from the London-based Friends of the Earth: "There are good grounds ... for being sceptical about the efficacy of 'population control' campaigns." There are no such campaigns, dear FoE, with the single exception of the Chinese Government's "two children" policy. Were you really so ignorant of what modern family planning is actually about?

Fortunately, even Friends of the Earth have recently moved away from their previous position, after a lot of work was done to educate and inform them. The big environmental organisations are still stuck mainly on the "avoidance" side of the argument but change is happening, although very slowly.

The leading broadcaster Sir David Attenborough, who has always refused to accept that consumption in rich countries is the only threat to the environment, has put it simply: "All our environmental problems become easier to solve with fewer people and harder – and ultimately impossible to solve – with ever more people." The leading environmental theorist Lester Brown has written extensively on the issues in *Full Planet, Empty Plates* and other books. Frederic Ballenegger, an environmental and ethical philosopher, argues: "Grossly unsustainable consumption patterns in the industrialized world, combined with uncontrolled demographic growth in the least developed countries and elsewhere, lead to the destruction of habitat and species, which is ethically indefensible ... Having acquired the means to destroy creation, humans also gained the duty to preserve it, including its diversity." The issues involved are also well described in a recent collection of essays by US environmentalists, *Beyond the Brink*.

In June 2012, at the Rio+20 Conference, a statement was issued by the combined non-governmental environmental organisations saying that "stable populations are an essential part of any sustainable future" and that "reducing our personal footprint does not help if we keep increasing the number of feet – we need to limit both." The United Nations Under-Secretary-General, Thoraya Ahmed Obaid, has added: "We cannot confront the massive challenges of poverty, hunger, disease and environmental destruction unless we address issues of population and reproductive health."

The International Union for Conservation of Nature and Natural Resources (IUCN), the world's largest and most diverse environmental network, has started to address the issue. Some important conservation organisations working in the most sensitive areas for wildlife are now introducing a health and family planning element for the people whose support they need if the programmes are to succeed. The Population and Sustainability Network is working to inform and involve environmentalists, to help them set up PHE projects, and to bring up the issues at key conferences. These are all steps in the right direction, but we need many more such moves before the environmental movement is fully committed to helping all women and men to plan for their children.

Can we look forward to a time when the environmental movement campaigns for women's rights to decide on their own fertility? We live in hope. But as my mother used to say, grimly, we die in despair. The optimistic view of this would be that the environmentalists – and international development specialists –

perhaps needed to go through a rejection of the old ideas of a "population explosion" focused purely on overall numbers, and come to a more humanitarian view that stresses the importance of enabling individual choices about having children, particularly for women. The same should of course go for the international women's movement. But it is a long time coming.

The opposition – the Global Gag advocates – are on a self-defined "crusade" to stop abortion and/or contraception. Well-meaning others are too ready to retreat in the face of such determination and aggression and their readiness to accuse others of advocating "population control", "eugenics" and the rest. Here then is perhaps the true explanation of the unwillingness of the international women's movement, the environmentalists and many development specialists to discuss fertility issues: it is the Adamants versus the Avoiders. The Adamants are aggressive, spoiling for a fight. The Avoiders are timid, careerist, and back away from confrontation.

While working on this, I am continually reminded of W B Yeats' lines from his poem "The Second Coming", written in 1919 during the build-up to the horrific civil war in Ireland:

"The best lack all conviction, while the worst
"Are full of passionate intensity."

We are not talking about a war, of course, unless you see this as a war on women. But the injuries, the suffering and loss of life from unwanted pregnancies and damaged mothers and babies are on an even greater scale. We should try to counter the "passionate intensity" of the fundamentalists and other Adamants with a conviction of our own that family planning is the ultimate lifesaver, and a key part of any work to relieve poverty and protect the environment on which we all depend.

Resources

Pope Francis, "Amoris Laetitia" ("Joy of Love") 2016.

Beth Holloway, "Circulatory Changes at Birth", URMC Online Medical Encyclopedia.

Michelle Goldberg, "The Means of Reproduction: Sex, Power, and the Future of the World" (Penguin Press, New York, 2009).

Diane J Horvath-Cosper, "Being a doctor who performs abortions means you always fear your life is in danger," *Washington Post,* 29 October 2015. Also various news reports in US news services and publications.

Troy Newman quoted in "Late-Stage Abortion Provider Won't Succumb to Protesters Who Forced Him Out of His Last Maryland Clinic," by Rachel M Cohen (The Intercept, online, 30 October 2017).

Germaine Greer, *Sex and Destiny: The Politics of Human Fertility* (HarperCollins, London, 1984).

Srilatha Batliwala, AWID Scholar Associate, "Beyond individual stories: women have moved mountains," Open Democracy website, 18 February 2013.

Angelika Arutyonova, "Starving the roots of women's human rights groups," Open Democracy website, 6 December 2013.

Martha Campbell, "Why the Silence on Population?" in Philip Cafaro and Eileen Crist (eds), *Life on the Brink: Environmentalists*

Confront Overpopulation (University of Georgia Press, US, 2012).

Paul R Ehrlich, "The Population Bomb", (Sierra Club and Ballantine Books, 1968, republished by Buccaneer Books, 1971). Anne Ehrlich was a co-author but omitted from the title after pressure from the publisher.

Lester R Brown, *Full Planet, Empty Plates: The new geopolitics of food scarcity* (W W Norton, 2012)

Philip Cafaro and Eileen Crist (eds), *Life on the Brink: Environmentalists Confront Overpopulation* (University of Georgia Press, 2012).

Frederic Ballenegger, "The Ethics and Theology of Population Dynamics," Harvard University Research Paper, December 2012.

Umbra Fisk, "Ask Umbra," in online environmental magazine *Grist*, 30 May 2016.

Interview with Roger Martin on *Grist*, 27 October 2011.

Chapter seven

ON THE WORLD STAGE
Adamants advance on governments

Never underestimate the power of organised religion when it is committed to a single project. This is certainly true of the Catholic Church, which has campaigned relentlessly to stop women and men choosing when to have children. Its campaign is not confined to its own members (about one in seven of the world's people) but seeks to impose this dogma on the whole world.

The vehicle for their influence is their pseudo-state, the Vatican. Its status is dubious, and its diplomatic presence worldwide is based on a fallacy that this is a State. The Vatican is now known internationally as the "Holy See", which is the official bureaucracy of this tiny area of Rome – smaller and less significant in reality than a small local authority. The Vatican itself is also a recent invention, not even a historical relic. It was created in 1929 by the Lateran Treaty between the Catholic Church and the then Italian head of state, the fascist leader Benito Mussolini.

Pope John Paul II, meeting there with Vladimir Putin in 2003, acknowledged: "What kind of state do I have here? You can see my whole state right from this window." Its total area is smaller than a standard-sized golf course. Unlike any national or even local authority it has no permanent residents, only church employees who leave when their contract is ended, and nobody who lives or works there has citizenship or voting rights. The Holy See/Vatican issues no passports except diplomatic ones. The area is inhabited almost entirely by men, most of whom have no wives or children. The very few women living and working there are mainly nuns, who are celibate and also have no children. If any children are born to people living there they have to be citizens of another country. There is no democratically elected government or local authority. Many of the basic municipal functions are carried out by the Government of Italy and municipality of Rome, including water and sewage, power supplies and rubbish collection, policing of the area and prosecution of any crimes committed there. The Vatican has some decorative "Swiss Guards" – formerly a group of mercenaries but later committed by the Swiss Government to the Pope's exclusive use. They have largely ceremonial duties inside the area, their official function being to protect him and his cardinals personally rather than to control the Vatican as a whole.

The Holy See/Vatican are not able to meet the criteria for a State under the 1933 Montevideo Convention on the Rights and Duties of States, one of the requirements being a permanent population. It refuses to ratify many human rights treaties. Yet this strange entity has now managed to get its own unique place at the United Nations as a "non-member State Permanent Observer" with free access to almost all meetings and their documentation, a free pass to the Delegates' Lounge, other bars and offices in the building, and even its own office at UN headquarters in New York which no country's delegation has. The Holy See is the only religious organisation that is given the privileges of a member State at the United Nations. All other world religions have the status of non-governmental organisations, apart from the Islamic world, which is emulating the Catholics and starting up the ladder of accreditation, as we shall see later. With a large and very effective Holy See diplomatic corps operating at all international meetings and conferences, as well as behind the scenes, and with ambassadors accredited to 178 countries of the world, the Holy See/Vatican may not be a State, but it claims the privileges of a member State of the UN in order to operate as an extremely powerful and effective lobbying machine. That lobbying power is directed mainly at its opposition to the case for human rights including women's rights, and women's rights including the right to choose when or whether to have children.

Obviously, the Catholic Church and its Holy See/Vatican are not the only opponents of family planning, but their influence has been so great on so many levels, from individual to international, that they require particular scrutiny. That has been strangely lacking, partly perhaps because of their "holier than thou" aura and the reluctance of many international observers to criticise a religious organisation. Since much of the influence is wielded behind the scenes it can also be difficult to know exactly what its representatives are doing. At the same time, they are seen, especially in the UN specialised agencies, as a menacing force that can break the careers of any officials who oppose them and their particular agenda. They can also threaten the funding of agencies if they step out of line, especially by their influence on the US administration and Congress. There seems to be a reluctance among officials of the UN and its agencies to even discuss the issue, since you can never be sure who might be listening.

Use of the Holy See/Vatican status also means that its influence can grow as the United Nations and its agencies become increasingly dominant in determining social and economic development goals and practices. This means that the Catholic Church can effectively impose its doctrines on the more than six billion people around the world who are not members, as well as the estimated one billion who are – something no other religion is able to do. This is defiance of the church's own Declaration on Religious Freedom, which states that Catholics must respect the beliefs of people of other faiths, accept that others are acting in accordance with their own conscience, and avoid "any hint of coercion" in spreading their own religious faith and practices.

We have to accept that the Catholic Church has the right to proclaim its own doctrine to its own believers on the question of sexuality, women's rights, modern contraception and abortion. Whether church members abide by that is another matter – most of them do not, given the choice. We even have to recognise that as an issue of "infallibility", it is difficult for the current hierarchy to backtrack on their position, however wrong or even immoral it may be. That is also a matter for the Church as a whole.

However, it is ironic that the Catholic Church's doctrinal insistence on promoting births is more powerfully achieved at the political and international level than it is among its own members through the power of their moral authority and preaching. The hierarchy's influence within the church itself – priests, bishops, archbishops and cardinals – is overshadowed by the formidable force that is the Vatican's political strength and its diplomatic service. Here the opposition to protected sex is based on the most conservative interpretation of doctrine, built up largely through the hierarchy's preference for promoting its most hard-line adherents from the ranks of ordinary priests, and carried forward by powerful individual men who make this a particular personal cause. There are plenty of contradictions in the theological teachings, highlighted by Pope Benedict's guarded approval of condoms as a "first step" in the fight against AIDS, while at the same time the Holy See still opposes their inclusion in international anti-AIDS programmes. Despite Benedict's ruling, their use is still prohibited in the vast Catholic network of HIV/ AIDS treatment, although there are rumours of some staff there handing them out secretly.

It is an extraordinary situation, especially when we recall that the Catholic doctrine of opposition to contraception is an invention of the late 19th century, as we have seen, and nothing to do with original Church teachings from Christ himself. In this chapter we take a look at their use of lobbying power to block people's access to choice through family planning.

Uninvited guests

Now a fixture on the international scene, giving the appearance of something perhaps rooted in antiquity, the Holy See/Vatican's status is in fact a very recent invention, the product of clever manoeuvring from 1929 onwards. It intensified after the Second World War with the conclusion of the Concordat with Italy – then a more intensely Catholic country than now – and some hard bargaining in early negotiations about the future United Nations and especially its World Health Organisation.

Amazingly, there is absolutely no legal basis for the Holy See's present status at the United Nations, its specialised agencies and its development-related conferences: no resolution of the General Assembly or Security Council, and no record of any other decision. Its attempt to join the League of Nations between the wars was rejected and it reportedly "regretted its exclusion". This was largely due to scepticism about its claims to be a State, and the possibility that it would have undue influence on the votes of member States with mainly Catholic populations.

In 1944 the Holy See made tentative inquiries to the United States about the eligibility of "Vatican City" to join the future United Nations, and was told by the then Secretary of State, Cordell Hull, that "the Vatican would not be capable of fulfilling all the responsibilities of membership". However, Vatican City had been able to join the World Telegraph Union (now the International Telecommunications Union) and the Universal Postal Union before World War II, being able to print and sell its own postage stamps. When the United Nations was being set up after the war this was used to gain admission into UN meetings, although only as an observer.

In 1948 the Food and Agriculture Organisation of the UN (FAO) became the first specialised UN agency to grant "Holy See/Vatican City" the status of Permanent Observer to its conferences, and a few others followed with Vatican representatives attending meetings, sometimes by invitation but at other times without any formal accreditation. They had a particular interest in the World Health Organisation, which they had earlier threatened to undermine by setting up their own international Catholic health body if the WHO promoted family planning. As a result the WHO committed itself to excluding contraceptive services from its programmes, and is still unwilling to integrate family planning into its worldwide health programmes. Since the WHO is the critical agency dealing with health internationally, the impact of this failure has been substantial. The full story of this would be worth investigation by future researchers.

It was not until 1964 that the then Secretary-General of the United Nations, U Thant, accepted the Holy See's self-designation as a Permanent Observer to the UN itself. Since he would not have taken any major decisions without consulting the US and Soviet Union, and since the Soviets may not have had a position on it, the Americans in particular were certainly instructing him to move in that direction.

In 2004 the Holy See was granted the right to speak freely in all debates, the right of reply to any other interventions, and the right to have their own documents circulated to all member States. There is no record of the General Assembly or the Security Council making any such decision. It was a back-door deal, with the conservative Catholic bishops' lobby using their influence with the United States Government to leverage a presence at the heart of the United Nations. The President in 2004 was George W Bush, and 2004 – interestingly – was his mid-term election year. It was an ideal opportunity for the bishops to extract concessions from him as the price of their support for his re-election, with no publicity and no political price to be paid domestically.

According to the UN's International Law Commission, "... observers were accepted only from non-member States which were full members of one or more specialized agencies and were generally recognized by Members of the United Nations." Since the Holy See's acceptance was never put to meetings of the members, this could not have been established. Interestingly, Pope John Paul II confirmed that the Holy See had not been invited into international bodies but had invited itself: "Pope Paul VI initiated the formal participation of the Holy See in the United Nations Organization."

This is critically important because of the use or abuse by the Holy See of its status at international meetings, especially those related to international development, human rights and specifically the rights of women. Unlike all other Observers at the UN, the Holy See is now automatically invited by the Secretariat to attend UN conferences and participate with "all the privileges of a State", even including the supposed right to vote, even though there is no basis for this in international law. The Holy See has used this situation relentlessly: as Catholics for Choice point out, "The official documents from UN conferences on women and population and development are replete with objections to the majority consensus made by representatives of the Holy See." They are also experts at the small print and will challenge even the slightest reference to women's rights, especially the right to sexual health and family planning.

Much of the influence wielded by the Vatican and Holy See, especially in the early days, was achieved by lobbying officials, delegations and individual governments, rather than submitting to votes by member States, and there is no doubt that this is still continuing. Stephen Mumford reveals that, at the International Population Conference in Mexico City in 1984, the Vatican achieved its goals through the United States delegation, which was made up largely of conservative Catholics appointed by then President Ronald Reagan. The US delegation took the official Vatican policy on abortion and family planning and helped to impose it on the meeting. This was followed by the key Cairo Conference in 1994, when the US delegation was more broadly based and no longer represented the hierarchy's position. The Vatican then had to come out from behind the screens and act in its own case. Everyone was stunned when the Holy See managed to shut down the whole meeting for its first six days. They then proceeded to challenge and obstruct every attempt to introduce the right to family planning. In desperation, the Chair of the meeting suspended discussions and, against all the usual procedures, invited representatives of all the non-governmental organisations present onto the conference floor to speak to the delegates.

At the 1995 Beijing Conference on Women, large sections of the final report had to be put in brackets (meaning they were not approved by consensus) even though State representatives had all agreed it. The Holy See had objected to these provisions, including the entire section on health, claiming that the text gave "totally unbalanced attention to sexual and reproductive health" and condemning family planning as "morally unacceptable". They were able to use their illegitimate position within the conference to veto decisions reached by representatives of all the world's governments.

How did we come to this?

Those of us who are not Catholics – the great majority of the world's people – should never accept that the church, via the Holy See, has the right to invite itself into the United Nations without any legal basis, to exploit their access to the maximum and to root around every document, every debate and every decision in order to block family planning and the women's rights agenda as a whole. They should not be dedicating their diplomatic and lobbying machine to this, nor funding it, nor putting pressure on the UN and specialised agency secretariats, individuals and governments. In short, they should call off the attack dogs and focus on their legitimate missions of justice and peace, leading moral campaigns on the international stage against poverty and war, and for human rights across the world. Yet the hierarchy has run out of control on this. They already have this UN status, they exploit it to the full, and it could be difficult to dislodge them. It will probably be up to governments to confront them officially on this, but in the meantime it is important for us to make it more widely known.

The Holy See machine does not just operate in international organisations, important though these are. Many countries with strong Catholic identities have been subjected to extreme pressure from the hierarchies in their own countries to block family planning, women's rights and even sex education. The Philippines has just recently emerged from decades of the bitterest battles with the Catholic bishops finally to pass a Reproductive Health Bill in 2013. The same is true of Ireland, where the Church has controlled social and health policy even though it was funded by the Irish State to provide the services. The result has been excessive levels of sickness, disability and death, which are unacceptable in any modern country. In 2012, for example, a desperately ill woman in Galway was allowed to die after she was refused a termination on the grounds that "this is a Catholic country" – although this was in a State hospital and not one of the many private Catholic ones.

Almost the whole of Latin America is still in the grip of these battles. Michelle Goldberg offers a detailed description of Catholic bishops' pressure on the governments of Costa Rica and Nicaragua, and its devastating effects for many women. The continent-wide network of liberal Catholic groups, Catolicas por el Derecho a Decidir (Catholics for the Right to Decide), issued a statement "stained by indignation and sadness" describing "the profound desire of a masculine church that feels the right to decide and choose what women want or should do with their lives," and in particular a model of the ideal woman whose mission has to include sacrifice, suffering and passivity. The emergence of the Zika virus with its devastating effects on foetuses, especially in Brazil, has highlighted the issue even more as women are denied contraception and safe abortion, and are forced to bear babies with microcephaly (undeveloped brains) and other severe birth defects. Countries most in need of family planning are at crisis point. Dr Vincent DeGennaro, who runs a women's health clinic in Haiti, told a reporter from *The Guardian*: "When we are in clinic and we offer women access to birth control they accept it like a hungry man eating food. We are failing women, and with the low cost of contraception, it's hard to say it's not deliberate." Giselle Carino of IPPF has commented: "The unfinished sexual and reproductive health and rights agenda has now become a humanitarian crisis in Latin America." The World Health Organisation has developed a Zika strategic response plan that would include family planning and education, but the $122m required to put it into practice was simply not there.

Backwards in the United States

Catholic bishops and the hierarchy generally have a strange hold over the United States federal government, even though Catholics are only a fifth of the US population, at most. This government in turn has a particularly powerful voice in the UN system, as a superpower and the largest UN contributor and aid donor in the world, but also because the headquarters of the United Nations itself, several specialised agencies, World Bank and IMF are on its territory and within its cultural atmosphere, including the American media. At the same time it gives and (for long periods) withholds big financial contributions to the UN itself and its specialised agencies, often because of opposition to the funding allocations in Congress but more recently ordered by President Trump. The dead hand of US on/off contributions creates artificial crises within these organisations, while also demanding various policy restrictions on their activities. Because of the separation of powers entrenched in its Constitution, and almost permanent election cycles, the US is peculiarly susceptible to special interest lobbying, especially on foreign affairs. Given enough single-mindedness, skilled lobbyists, a lot of money and a large and well-organised membership, US government policy can be turned in a particular direction quite easily. The Catholic lobby can exert powerful pressure on the President, House of Representatives and Senate, often by threatening that Catholics, their orders and organisations will withdraw election funding and urge their members to vote them out if they do not follow an ultra-conservative line.

This was certainly achieved by the US Catholic bishops with President Richard Nixon. In 1969, Nixon accepted that family planning was critical to the world's wellbeing and said in a message to Congress, "When future generations evaluate the record of our time, one of the most important factors in their judgment will be the way in which we respond to population growth. Let us act in such a way that those who come after us – even as they lift their eyes beyond Earth's bounds – can do so with pride in the planet on which they live, with gratitude to those who lived on it in the past, and with continuing confidence in the future." It was a remarkable statement but anathema to the bishops, and within five years his Administration was in full retreat on this issue.

In 1970, Nixon had created the Commission on Population Growth and the American Future, which after two years of study made more than 70 recommendations. They included making contraception and safe abortion available for all who needed them, if necessary at governments' expense. However, 1972 was a presidential election year and Nixon became convinced that the Catholic bishops would be able to swing the balance of voting against him. He completely abandoned the report even though he had himself commissioned it, and none of the recommendations was ever adopted. In 1974 he had another try, ordering all agencies of the federal government through National Security Study Memorandum 200 (NSSM 200) to determine the "implications of world population growth". However, by the time it reported in 1975 he had been forced to resign and was succeeded by President Ford, who did not pursue it.

The report concluded that continued rapid population growth posed a risk to "world economic, political, and ecological systems and, as these systems begin to fail, to our humanitarian values". It also stated that "population factors are indeed critical in, and often determinants of, violent conflict in developing areas" including both civil wars and regional conflicts. They could weaken unstable governments and "open the way to extremist regimes". It recommended that "developing countries make family planning information, education and means available to all their peoples by 1980" with the United States contributing financially and offering medical and technical support. Again the US Catholic bishops mobilised against it, adopting a plan to build a coalition against these proposals, which involved the extreme right across the country. The NSSM 200 report, although endorsed by President Ford, was never published and became a classified document. Under President Reagan, whose top team included a high proportion of conservative Catholics, the Administration agreed to alter its foreign aid programme to incorporate an outright "global gag" ban on the use of its aid funds if they included any help for birth control or abortion. Officials of the US Agency for International Development (AID) were sent to Rome for long discussions with the Holy See, and were finally forced to reverse many of their programmes. All funding was cut off for the International Planned Parenthood Federation (IPPF) and UN Fund for Population Activities. During the Bush years, funding was also withheld for UN Children's Fund (Unicef) to help street children and families in extreme poverty.

This in turn has had a profoundly inhibiting effect on the United Nations, its agencies and the international development scene. Other countries, especially in Europe, have made up some of the shortfall in funding from the US, but until recently were unable to match the amounts involved. Even under President Obama, although some funding was restored, the commitment to family planning was still less than previous levels, and a restrictive Helms Amendment on abortion continued to block any help – real or imagined – for safe abortion. The Trump administration has now returned to the gag rule, slashed funding, and is now planning to divert aid money to groups that are spreading false information about family planning or advocating abstinence from sex. Far from combatting terminations, which is the stated aim, this greatly increases the numbers of unwanted pregnancies and dangerous attempts at abortion.

New alliances

Although the overall pattern of Holy See/Vatican activity has been ultra-conservative, there was a period, while there were debates around the Pontifical Commission on Birth Control and the 1968 *Humanae Vitae* edict, when the Holy See looked as if it might take a more charitable view. I was at an international development conference in 1970 where there was a delightful Holy See representative whose favourite expression was "Down with the Pill!" Certainly no such jokes would be allowed now from their representatives. The ultra-conservatives are firmly in charge of the Catholic hierarchy, and particularly its international "diplomatic" operations. Their most recent tactic is to establish a coalition of ultra-conservative elements – including fundamentalists of other religions – against women's rights.

The Islamic world has been well aware of the privileged position of the Holy See/Vatican at international meetings, and their conservatives want a piece of the action for themselves. The United Nations organisation, if it was not prepared to challenge the Holy See claims, could hardly refuse this new demand. The result is the Permanent Delegation of the Organisation of Islamic Cooperation (OIC) to the UN Offices in Geneva and Paris. Since there is no single body representing all Muslims, this is something cobbled together for international representation and is likely only to pursue the most conservative version of an Islamic view of the world, and also one which wholly or largely excludes Muslim women's views. It still has much less access to international debates than the Holy See/Vatican, but this move does mean getting a foot on the international ladder. It also means they can more easily co-ordinate the more conservative governments of Islamic countries to speak and vote against measures they oppose. Other conservative religious organisations could follow with fresh demands for their own representation at the UN, its conferences and its development agencies.

The OIC have already joined forces with the Holy See at specialised UN conferences to oppose people's access to contraception. At the 2012 "Rio+20" Earth Summit on sustainable development, for example, all reference to "reproductive rights" was rigorously excluded from the final text, and no recognition of the link between family planning and international development was allowed into the document. The notion of women's rights overall was also firmly excluded, despite the advocacy of women's and family planning organisations:

many were excluded from the meeting as not being delegates of member States, and they were overcome by a tiny minority of implacable opponents, led by the Holy See, including the representatives of the Philippines, Argentina, Malta and Egypt. In that same year a proposed UN declaration on the rights of women, including an end to domestic violence and marital rape, was opposed by delegations from the Holy See, Russia, Pakistan, Iran and Syria. At that time Egypt was governed by the Muslim Brotherhood, which claimed that the declaration would lead to the "complete disintegration of society".

The case of Russia opposing women's rights seems anomalous, but it is consistent with its support and even finance for ultra-conservative groups in other countries, including the Front Populaire in France, the Trump election campaign in the US, and the Brexit campaign in the UK. One commentator observed: "There is a belief that Russia is simply trying to flex its political muscle in the international sphere to show that it is a force to be reckoned with." In other words there is an element of mischief here, an anti-democracy stance which uses the ultra conservatives in the West as its chosen instrument – the mirror image of the old Communist International (Comintern) perhaps. The Russian Orthodox Church is also increasingly influential in the country and its leadership has been condemning contraception and abortion, while also – astonishingly – opposing moves to combat violence against women. The Orthodox Church leader, Patriarch Kirill, who met the Catholic Pope for the first time in 2016, has even claimed that "feminism could destroy Russia".

On the international scene the Russian Government's influence has also tended to silence some countries, including Cuba and Ecuador, which see Russia as an ally on other issues. In the otherwise progressive European block of countries, Poland, Malta and Hungary – all with ultra-conservative governments – have also reversed their previous support for women's rights. Women, it seems, are becoming disposable, a bargaining chip within national and international politics. If a government has domestic problems with religious fundamentalists, then cheap concessions can be made in the international forums on women and especially access to contraception, in the hope of boosting support at home and within their regional grouping.

The conservative eugenic movement in the United States is highly organised and heavily funded. It links up with other conservative movements across the world even if they seem to be at opposite extremes in terms of politics or religion. For this purpose they quietly downplay their claims made to a home audience that Americans and Europeans will be "swamped" by Muslims and other "races", and instead emphasise a supposed common worldwide interest in keeping women and families under male authority and made to keep "breeding".

Among their activities, reported in detail by Michelle Goldberg, has been a series of international meetings such as the one organised by the US-funded World Congress of Families in Warsaw in 2007, which brought together thousands of conservatives from the US, Poland, the Vatican and around the world, including Catholics, Mormons, Eastern Orthodox and evangelical Christians as well as some Muslim and Jewish people. Organiser Allan Carlson, a right wing Protestant, urged delegates to promote childbirth wherever possible, telling the meeting: "Sexual radicals would twist and distort the procreative act, turning it away from the creation of new life. Neo-Malthusians would accelerate the disappearance of nations and the depopulation of the earth."

Following the Islamist terror attack on the World Trade Center on 9/11 the World Congress of Families cut formal ties with Muslim conservatives but, according to Carlson, continued on a much more informal but still very effective basis, and they continued to befriend individual delegates to UN meetings and conferences. Meanwhile, under the Bush and Trump administrations the US Government has also put powerful pressure on governments to fall into line when voting at the UN. They have not hesitated to suggest that US aid programmes in their countries might be affected if their delegates vote the "wrong" way.

Problematic combinations

At recent UN conferences some delegates have been observed following the Holy See's line against women's reproductive rights, even though it contradicted the pro-choice policies pursued in the countries they are supposed to represent. The governments of many smaller countries do not have sophisticated systems of briefing their delegates and issuing instructions during meetings - their capabilities are a small fraction of the Holy See's diplomatic service which can call in extra people to enforce the official line whenever women's rights are being debated. The largely all-male delegations from smaller countries are able to revert to their own personal prejudices about women, or can be persuaded by well-funded lobbyists to follow a conservative line, especially on issues which are presented to them as the defence of "our tradition" even when this contradicts the policies of their own governments.

Margaret Owen, a veteran of UN meetings who represents widows internationally, summed up the deteriorating situation at these meetings in a 2013 report on the Commission on the

Status of Women: "States are now regrouping in problematic combinations – for women's reproductive rights – to show their strength and muscle." She particularly cited disappointment that the delegation from Bangladesh "that led, for years in the South Asia region, on family planning services and programmes, that targeted hard-to-reach women, should have now wandered to the other side."

She paints a picture of closeted delegates making their decisions in the main building while six women from non-governmental organisations were "talking mostly to each other in the 'ghetto' of the Church Centre, that lies across the road from the UN building," discussing topics like torture and rape, genital mutilation, criminal trafficking, acid- attacks and other violence against women. With limited access to observer passes, and no speaking rights, many had been excluded from the UN building itself. Meanwhile the Holy See delegation is able to use complex manoeuvres and heavy lobbying of conservatives of other delegations inside and outside the conference hall and in the corridors and tea-rooms, not only to block new rights for women but even to weaken the texts previously agreed on the subject.

There seems to be an element of apathy creeping into the debates. One initiative after another for women's rights, against sexual violence, for homosexual rights and especially for reproductive rights is being blocked and even pushed back by these growing alliances of ultra-conservatives, led by the Holy See. There can be a strong feeling that the battles are just not worth it – or that the only people who can fight them are a handful of mainly western, developed countries, which keep pressing for a rights agenda. They are rights that can so easily be blocked by a single opponent, and now by the growing alliances of the Catholics, Islamists and ultra-conservatives even from countries whose policies are solid.

The result of all these processes is that, despite meeting after meeting on women's rights, reproductive rights and sustainable development, the UN system, with its specialised agencies, is still having to base its actions on the 1994 Cairo Conference on Population and Development (ICPD). Where there have been bold declarations in favour of family planning, as with the first Regional Conference on Population and Development for Latin America and the Caribbean in 2013, the negotiations were led mostly by experts (whether from Ministries of Women or Health) and not by the Ministries of Foreign Affairs which continue to dominate most of the UN meetings and which are not in touch with the real issues on the ground.

The one major achievement recently has been the incorporation of family planning into the Sustainable Development Goals of 2015, a triumph which reversed the Holy See's successful blocking of this element from the previous Millennium Development Goals of 2001. Goal 3.7 of the new SDGs reads: "By 2030, ensure universal access to sexual and reproductive health-care services, including for family planning, information and education, and the integration of reproductive health into national strategies and programmes." Goal 5.6 reads: "Ensure universal access to sexual and reproductive health and reproductive rights." These clauses were achieved with an almost superhuman effort by governmental and non-governmental organisations. One battle won: so many more to go.

As long as the agenda for family planning is set in terms of human rights and especially women's rights, I suggest, it will be an uphill battle in international conferences. This is why, in the next chapter, I suggest that we focus not on rights, but on needs.

Resources

Catholics for Choice, "The Catholic Church at the United Nations: Church or State?", Washington DC, 2013. ISBN: 978-1-936421-05-3. Catholics for Choice have a "See Change" campaign to challenge the Holy See's representation at the UN.

Stephen D Mumford, "The Vatican's Role in the World Population Crisis: the untold story," presentation to Main Line Unitarian Church, 1996 (Center for Research on Population and Security, 1996).

Michelle Goldberg, *The Means of Reproduction: Sex, Power and the Future of the World* (Penguin Press, New York, 2009).

Derek S Hoff, *The State and the Stork: The population debate and policy making in US history (University of Chicago Press, 2012).*

Stephen D Mumford, "The Life and Death of NSSM 200: How the destruction of political will doomed a U.S. population policy," (Amazon.com, 1996).

Carl Bernstein, "The US and the Vatican on Birth Control," *Time* magazine, 24 February 1992.

PART FOUR: THE SOLUTIONS

Chapter eight

A NEW WAY FORWARD
It's the poverty, stupid

In the richer countries modern contraception is now almost universal, and has benefitted everybody either directly or indirectly. Good family planning is one reason these countries have become so much richer than the rest of the world. Over the last century it has enormously improved women's and children's health and survival prospects, causing death rates to come down with astonishing speed. It is only two or three generations ago that women were forced to bear children they did not want, where many were injured or died in childbirth or from illegal and dangerous abortions, where child mortality was high and where the only answer to the "surplus" population was to emigrate to every other continent in the world with all the long-term disruption and conflict that resulted. With the large settler populations still remaining in some countries, this still continues to this day.

Family size in developed countries is now largely in line with what parents want and can support. Women have entered higher education in very large numbers and have now become an integral part of the workplace, contributing to household and national income and gaining personal autonomy and a large degree of equality with men. Nobody would claim there are no problems left for women in these countries, but the progress in terms of health and welfare has been astonishing.

This also means that most countries of Europe, North America and Australasia have a generally stable population, which, although distorted by birth "bulges", especially after World War II, is well on the way to becoming balanced between people of different ages. The main source of any population growth in the West now is immigration and not births. If the worst they can find to worry about is our attractiveness to migrants, or our improved life expectancy and a supposedly "ageing population" then we have come a very long way.

This is now perhaps the biggest difference between rich and poor countries: we have modern contraception and they, on the whole (with some notable exceptions) do not – or only for the privileged few. At the moment, on the international scene, double standards rule: that modern contraception is not important, or is even dangerous for "them" but not for "us". Some are claiming that it is a cultural imposition – for "them" but not for "us". It is double standards all the way.

The same human needs should be recognised everywhere. We should value the development and equality potential of the family planning services that have so benefitted the richer countries and extend them to the poorer ones. Wealthier people cannot justify having it all, but not allowing others to have it when they need it. We should not tolerate the gulf between richer countries, where people can make critical life decisions about pregnancy and children, and poorer ones where they do not have the means to make these decisions but can too easily be overwhelmed by random life events.

A campaign to equalise access to decision-making between rich and poor countries and people is a much better way forward than campaigning under the banner of "sexual and reproductive rights". As we have seen in the last chapter, the SRHR case has been repeatedly beaten back by the Catholic hierarchy, together with fundamentalists and nationalists in different countries. Their growing alliances mean that they can prevent SRHR from becoming a universally accepted mainstream agenda. The Vatican/Holy See, alongside ultra-conservative and autocratic governments in the Islamic world and elsewhere, have built an increasing resistance to any talk of women's rights or even "human rights" generally, to the point where any mentions become taboo. They are carrying out almost a military-style "search and destroy" operation on any mention or hint of women's rights that might relate to decisions about children. Even if Pope Francis is able to reduce the ferocity and the funding, the opposition is entrenched and there is no prospect of this changing any time soon.

We need a tactical change of approach. Human rights are critical to the international agenda, and so is family planning, but attaching the two together is a dead end. Where our side has won important battles, like incorporating reproductive choice into the recent Strategic Development Goals, there will be a constant battle to ensure that this is funded on the scale that is required to meet the needs, while other SDGs may get most of the money and the effort.

The case for arguing needs instead of rights – especially for women and children – is that basic needs are universal. Rights (whether we like it or not) can be subject to different cultural and legal environments. Despite the enormous international efforts to achieve a universal standard of human rights, especially over the last 70 years, these are under constant challenge from reactionaries. That battle must go on, but we do not have the time to wait for it to be won. The case for choosing the numbers and timing of children has to be pursued separately, and as a matter of urgency. We have to support the choices that will help people move out of the vicious circle of poverty, hunger and illness. The UN calculates that 36 million die of hunger and malnutrition every year – a person every second, mostly women and children. Unintended births are a contributor to this horror. We have to show that this is unacceptable in a world trying to end poverty and promote inclusion.

I suggest too that it would be better for the universal human rights agenda if people's decisions about children were removed from that debate. The fight for human rights must go on, of course – the right to life, to freedom from torture and the right to family life. Women's rights in general – against rape and domestic violence, against genital mutilation, against trafficking and exploitation – also need to be part of the human rights agenda. But the contentious issues around family planning should be discussed separately from rights if either agenda is to make real progress.

In addition to that, the term "Sexual and Reproductive Health and Rights" (SRHR) confronts further resistance because of the reference to sexuality. Not only is women's sexuality a forbidden topic for many conservative societies and governments, but the SRHR banner also incorporates the rights of lesbians and gay men, bisexuals and transsexuals as well as questioning and intersex. That agenda is also very important but it should be tackled separately and not as an add-on to SRHR. Otherwise the anti-gay backlash starts to overlap with the anti-choice one, and a proper discussion becomes obscured and overlaid with the sometimes hysterical reaction from conservatives to either or both.

As for the family planning advocates, it is time to find new ways forward that do not depend on arguments about "rights". We have seen an irresistible force (us) confronted by an immovable object (them) and the result is that we have been bashing our collective heads against a brick wall of refusal that is simply being built higher and higher. We need more sophisticated tactics, which would mean we sidestep that wall, making their arguments about their dogma or "culture" as irrelevant as the medieval disputes within the Catholic Church about how many angels could stand on the head of a pin. How would it look if they started opposing motions for better health for all, including maternity and newborn health and survival? Let us abandon "rights" versus "culture" and go for the universal needs of all people everywhere.

A new language of needs

If we want to gain momentum on this issue we should be embedding it in the drive against poverty and speaking the language of basic needs: the universal human need for food and water to sustain life, the need for good health and the need for the right number of children to ensure women's survival and wellbeing as well as health and welfare for their children and families. We should stress also the need to incorporate all of these children into stable families and communities: no more unwanted children, or "surplus" adults with no prospect of a livelihood and no place in their own society. Just as we need food, water and shelter, and a community to belong to, we also need the right number of children to take the family forward, sustaining and hopefully increasing these resources.

We should not forget, either, the need to preserve our natural environment – fresh water, viable agricultural land and fisheries, an ecological balance with forests, grasslands and seas. We also have to address the proliferating conflicts over water resources, whether local or national, which increasing numbers of people bring. However, this is not about nations or numbers but individuals, families and communities. Our focus has to be on individual and family decision-making, based on individual and family needs.

Women and families living in poverty need the right number of children to secure their own and their children's health and wellbeing. An unexpected, unwanted pregnancy can often tip the balance from survival to disaster. Family resources that are enough to meet the basic needs of life and health for all its members would often become inadequate if there were an addition to the family. Even worse is the loss or ill health of a mother, which is happening with deadly regularity and is a disaster for many families in poor communities. Children without a mother may end up abandoned, homeless and with the most dismal future. Orphans may often be brought into the family of a sister, grandmother or other relative, who may already be struggling to provide enough food for their existing children and, by sharing it out more thinly, will end up with not enough food, let alone education or the prospect of a livelihood when they grow up. Without modern contraception, and good maternity care, there can be no way out of extreme deprivation and personal suffering for hundreds of millions of people. The enormous numbers of women going for illegal abortions, knowing just how dangerous they are, and that they risk death as a result, is proof enough of women's need for safe and effective contraception.

Younger women and girls need to avoid pregnancy when they are already having sex but their bodies are too immature to bear children safely. Millions are facing this whether through forced or child marriage, from sexual violence, through the "sugar daddy" system of sex with an older and wealthier man, or of course through consensual sex with other young people. Women building up a livelihood, whether as employees or as independent farmers or traders, may need a period without pregnancy in order to establish themselves. Those who already have one or more children may need a respite from pregnancy to allow their bodies to recover fully, and to feed and care for their existing children. Those who are sick or malnourished may also need relief from the heavy demands of pregnancy. Women approaching the menopause may need the assurance that they will not have yet another child if they do not want that, if the family would suffer or if their health would be badly affected. At the same time there will also be women who find it hard to conceive, or to carry a pregnancy to term, and choice about children should be available for them too.

This would not be complete without discussing abortion as an essential element in family planning, a backup if contraception fails. At the moment the debate is between "pro-choice" and "pro-life". The distinction needs to be revised. Without legal and safe abortion, huge numbers of women resort to illegal and highly dangerous abortions, which endanger their lives and, in too many cases, cause their deaths. Abortions are at epidemic levels in those countries that have made them illegal, especially if there is no easy access to contraception. Hospital facilities which should be devoted to maternity and infant care are struggling to cope with women suffering from the catastrophic effects of these abortions. This is even reported to be happening in the United States where, although it is legal, persistent attacks have closed many clinics so that legal abortions are too far away or too expensive for the women most in need.

There is one slogan used by campaigners that is crucial to this: "Keep it legal, keep it safe." Nobody can stop abortion: it is universal and inevitable. The way to reduce the numbers is by the best possible contraception. The only way to save women's lives from dangerous abortion is to make it legal. This has to be the cornerstone of any defence of legal abortion. It is not pro-choice versus pro-life, pro-abortion versus anti-abortion. It is: stop the deaths of women (many of them already mothers) because of the attempts to stop legal and safe terminations, attempts that only increase dangerous abortion, especially among the poorest women.

Perhaps the slogan could be "Stop the *killer* abortions."

Sex and development

Sex is popular everywhere, but especially in poor communities where it costs nothing. It can be entertainment, pleasure and relaxation all in one. Where women get their own pleasure from sex, that is great. But we also have to recognise that far too often, sex is an obligation that can be imposed on women. It is important to be realistic about sex, especially in repressive relationships and societies where girls and women have little or no choice in the matter; some religious authorities order wives to allow their husbands to have sex at any time. Many of the religious moralisers who are so quick to condemn women who step out of line fail to understand that sexual violence and sexual obligation are also moral issues.

These moralisers are often content with sexual coercion since some of them get their own sexual gratification in this way. In policy terms they may see sexual freedom for men as a means to producing more and more children for their own benefit. They are remarkably quiet about telling other men to refrain from sexual violence, or from insisting on marriage without the woman's consent. If priests, imams and all the rest were to preach a real sexual morality for men as well as women we would have many fewer unwanted pregnancies and births. Are they perhaps unwilling to apply morality to men as they do to women? If condemnation is to be reserved for women only, you have to wonder whose religion this is and what kind of God they are imagining.

Their sometimes obsessive attention is directed at instructing others how to do it, when to do it, with whom, and damn the consequences in terms of pregnancy and future children. In the real world, sexuality is not subject to their rules: it is infinitely variable, subject to a complex variety of emotions, and quite often without thought for the future. Good sex, freely chosen, is better when there is no worry about pregnancy. Routine "good enough" sex needs contraception. Sex as an obligation or a business transaction, through rape or forced marriage, means women are in even greater need of it to preserve some element of control over their own bodies.

The Ugandan doctor Lydia Mungherera told Michelle Goldberg: "Women don't have rights in deciding when to have sex, and how to have sex – whether to use a condom or not. Men can have as many partners as they want, and women don't have a choice. You find that women are locked up in marriages where they're not happy, and they don't have the financial and educational empowerment to leave those marriages. There's a lot of domestic violence."

If we could be more realistic about what sex is really like for millions of women we could perhaps see that all sex requires protection from unwanted pregnancy.

Universal needs

Need is a powerful notion. We should embrace people's need to make their own life decisions, as a core element in any development process. We should be aware that the need for family planning also applies to men, since their interests in stable families are just as important, though perhaps less obvious. Introducing family planning services is also far more difficult if men are actively opposed, or not involved. Marriage and relationships are often far from perfect but for many men, their wives and partners are precious and irreplaceable. How sad it is when they see this only after their wife dies. Yet the biggest need of all belongs with the women themselves, and of course the children. All women need their health and strength not only for themselves, but in order to look after children and often other dependants – older or disabled – who may have nobody else to care for and support them.

This is the missing link in so many poverty eradication strategies. Nobody should pretend that family planning alone will solve all the problems of poverty (our opponents love to accuse us of saying it will). Without it, though, the battle will always be uphill, a never-ending struggle to contend with the downward forces of enforced sex and marriage for women, enforced pregnancies, and more children than they can safely bear or are able to care for.

It is the needs of individuals – women, men and children – that should always come first in this debate. Too often I hear both theorists and practitioners of development talk about "population" to address the growth in human numbers. Although we cannot avoid the use of the population concept, it is an argument that is going nowhere. It has become that unwanted, old, smelly dog, a toxic P-word in many international circles. I would like to rename the lovely UN Fund for Population as the UN Fund for People. "Population" is also addressing the issue from completely the wrong direction. We should not be advocating choice merely because the abstract concept of "population" demands it. We should be pressing for individual welfare and development through a greater ability to make life decisions. Individual and family needs should always be the focus if poverty itself is to be overcome.

Look after the people, and the population will take care of itself.

Cultures, governments and laws differ around the world, but human bodies remain the same everywhere. We need enough food, of good nutritional value, water and good enough health, wherever we are. Our capacity for reproduction is the same worldwide, and our need to control that is universal. Women's particular needs around sex, pregnancy, childbearing and child rearing are the same in any part of the world.

I am reminded of the famous speech by Shakespeare's Shylock in *The Merchant of Venice*, raging at his treatment as a Jew. Changing the text slightly: "I am a poor woman. Has not any woman eyes? has not any woman hands, organs, dimensions, senses, affections, passions? fed with the same food, hurt with the same weapons, subject to the same diseases, healed by the same means... If you prick us, do we not bleed? if you tickle us, do we not laugh? if you poison us, do we not die?"

Everybody's needs can be met if there are enough resources (water, food, housing, health care) and no discrimination in how they are distributed. The question of hugely unequal resources, which underlies all development, applies very much to choosing children: the more developed a country is, the more likely its people are to have that choice. The poorer it is (with some notable exceptions) the less likely to have any choice. Within each country, too, it is the poorest women who have the least choice, and with that the greatest risk of unwanted pregnancies, dangerous abortions, and a serious risk of death or serious disability for themselves and for their children. Family planning is essential to any moves to combat poverty.

It is too often claimed that women will adopt family planning when they become educated. In fact this has become a tired cliché of development. It is true that there is a correlation – women with education are likely to move out of the poorest category and have more choices as well as knowledge of what is available. However it is not true that poor women with little or no formal education will not adopt contraception. There are now many projects demonstrating this to be a rather patronising view of poor women, who are just as keen to make their own decisions about pregnancy as those with more money and education, once they have the chance. Many walk long distances to get their supplies of contraception.

A feature of many poor areas is that the women there have lost traditional methods of limiting pregnancies. These may include women's secret societies and rituals, including the initiation of young girls; sometimes the physical separation of new mothers and babies; extended periods of breast-feeding; and the use of techniques and especially medicinal herbs known to "wise women" in the community. Modern societies have tried to eliminate traditional forms of birth control, and women's knowledge and skills have been suppressed in some areas.

In Europe and the newly settled United States, in previous centuries, women with secret knowledge were branded as "witches", and many were tortured and killed. The cruelties involved in denying women choices about children are too often forgotten – including "traditional" ways of neglecting or killing unwanted babies, especially if they are girls, or born with disabilities. Modern medicine and science allow us all to move past these horrors and regulate births in safer and more effective ways. It offers a shift towards a more humane tradition.

The process of modernisation or westernisation, which is contained within "development", has since colonial times altered the balance of power and influence between women and men. This has been very much to the disadvantage of the women, who have been losing their autonomy and their own real traditions, and made to accept the men's version of what "our tradition" is about. Cultures are dynamic, and traditions too are constantly evolving. Let the women decide what is right for them and their communities, and find a balance of old and new traditions that are healthy for everyone.

Writing as a woman in a developed country, I have relied on contraception to enable good health and a life I have decided for myself, within or outside relationships. It has enabled me to choose the right number of children for me (in my case, none) which I hope is of benefit to society. I want that possibility to be available to all women everywhere, no matter what their personal circumstances or obligations. We now have the means to offer contraception and early abortion, which is safe and effective, in any area of any country in the world: something that has never existed before. All we need are the resources.

Individuals, governments and international development

The list of governments that have understood and promoted birth control options for their people is surprising. One of the poorest countries in the world, Bangladesh, has instituted wide-ranging programmes, with the support of international agencies and voluntary aid groups. One of the countries most recently torn by civil conflict, Rwanda, has done the same. One of the most strictly Islamic, Iran, has made it a high priority. Poverty and conflict do not prevent enlightened thinking by governments. They can be the reason it becomes critical to moving forward.

Yet many other governments around the world still use these factors as an excuse. "More children, and yet more!" is their mantra. It is numbers they want, not better lives – quantity and not quality of life – and they will use "our culture" as an excuse. Numbers for cannon fodder, for child labour, for perceived advantage in sectarian conflicts, as members of their religion or ethnic group in competition with others, or even as voters to keep them comfortably in power – sometimes to use the resources of the state to enrich themselves, their families and their loyal associates. They then wonder why there is so much poverty, so many homeless children, youth unemployment, crime, mass migrations, environmental destruction and burning of wild areas, warlords and terrorist groups, and vicious armed conflicts. They fail to understand why "economic development" is not happening, or why there is deepening poverty among so many individuals and communities.

Governments and the international community are unanimous in wanting economic development. They also, of course, want peace and stability. Yet this cannot happen while so many people are subject to life events – births, deaths, illness and disability, debt and dependency, loss of land or animals, environmental disasters – with no possibility of deciding whether or when to have more children in that situation. An unwanted pregnancy can be the disaster that pushes whole families back into deep poverty, and a dangerous abortion can be their only way of trying to avert that disaster. To have any chance at all of improving their lives, health and welfare, people living in poverty need to be able to make these crucial life decisions for themselves. In areas where there is no modern family planning provision at all, people do not even believe it is possible. It is only when there is a safe and effective programme that they will gain the confidence that will enable them to take control.

We are not talking of the impossible. It has been estimated that if half of all women had one less child, population growth would stop and our numbers would be stable.

Governments around the world hold the key to effective action. The international effort to bring modern contraception is long on experience and expertise, but very short on finance. The only UN agency offering any funds is the UN Fund for Population (UNFPA), which has very limited resources. Programmes are at crisis point. It is worth noting that the "Brexit" vote in Britain was considered a blow to international contraceptive programmes. The reason? Britain has been one of the biggest supporters, through its aid programme, and the fall in the pound following that vote meant 10% less money in dollars for family planning. With Trump in power in the US, there are savage cuts, attempts at a "global gag" and certainly little or no increase in funds for family planning as stand-alone projects and programmes. There will be no new money and probably a cut to existing programmes. The only way forward is for all aid bodies to integrate this into their own programmes and budgets, either offering family planning services themselves or partnering with organisations that are already doing it.

Family planning should be integral to fighting poverty, not some separate activity. Governments of the poorer countries also need to start taking a lead, putting this higher up their list of priorities for their own funds and requests for international assistance. Support and expertise from the international community will be there if new sources of funding can be found.

Health

One of the causes of poverty – which is also a cause of great suffering – is the failure to ensure that all people have access to quality healthcare without being expected to pay large amounts of cash for it. An estimated 150 million people each year are pushed into poverty, or further into poverty, because they have to pay high costs for healthcare when there is illness or injury. And 400 million people do not have access to the most basic health services. For many national governments, funding for health is not a priority. A recent report from the World Health Organization (WHO) shows that between 2000 and 2014, public funding for health from domestic sources in low and middle-income countries stagnated. The international target is for governments to spend 5% of their GDP on basic health care, with international donors supplementing this with carefully targeted interventions that do not replace national funding.

One of the features of development economics is the disregard for people's health as an element in transforming poverty into self-sufficiency. In cost-benefit analysis, it gets very low or even zero recognition. Development economists have a very crude understanding of the benefits of contraception in particular, and this distorts their calculations. I have heard one economist, for example, claiming that it is not cost-effective to give contraception to a woman nearing the menopause because "she has already done her environmental damage". This kind of thinking is crude and offensive. It also fails to take account of the influence of older women on younger ones in deciding whether or not to use contraception.

International organisations need to change their thinking, with health not only taking a higher priority by incorporating family planning as an essential element. Ask the World Bank, IMF or UNDP about this and until now they would have little to say: they may merely suggest that health promotion and/or family planning be added as an optional extra to major country investments.

This is starting to change, for example in 2016 with a $500 million World Bank International Development Association credit to Nigeria for a "Saving One Million Lives" initiative for maternal and child health. The indicators for success here will include contraceptive prevalence as well as maternal and child health and survival rates. This kind of programme needs to be rolled out to many more countries. Until personal health is added into the development equation, with family planning as an essential element, any economic and social progress will be limited and limiting. Meanwhile, the specialised UN agencies, like the World Health Organisation and the UN Children's Fund (Unicef) in particular, also need a radical overhaul without fear of retaliation from the US and other funders, so as to direct their own funds towards help with family planning as an essential element in health promotion. There can be no real health or welfare without choice. This is an investment, not a cost: the UN's Global Strategy for Women's, Children's and Adolescents' Health (2016) shows that almost a quarter of income growth in low- and middle-income countries between 2000 and 2011 resulted from improved health outcomes.

This is yet another area where services we can take for granted in most of the richer countries – a health service that is there when we need it – is simply absent in most developing nations, especially among the poorest countries and the poorest of their people.

There is no development without health, and no health without family planning.

Wanted babies?

The gap between rich and poor – countries and individuals – is not just about money. It is also about the decision-making gap, where the richer you are the more control you have over your own life and that of your children and other family members. This control means you are much less likely to get overwhelmed by those random life events that happen to all of us: illness, accidents, pregnancy or having to care for family and friends when they need it. Without choices it is like being in rough seas that can destroy your fragile boat when there is nobody to rescue you if it overturns, or to tow you safely towards the harbour.

Birth control will not, by itself, solve all the problems of poverty. Without it, though, those problems will only get worse. If family planning is combined with initiatives in the media, alongside better health services in poor areas and campaigns against child marriage, child sex and premature childbearing, other forced marriage, and female genital mutilation, the outcome for people now living in poverty can be transformative. The many successful projects in many parts of the world are now demonstrating just this.

Babies should be precious. They should be wanted and needed. Babies are our present and our key to the future. Let us have sex without the worry of unwanted pregnancy. Let us all decide whether to have babies, and when is the right time in our lives to give them the best possible childhood and the best future as adults. These are the biggest life decisions that anyone can make, and we should all be able to make these decisions for ourselves, for our communities and for our world.

Resources

Michelle Goldberg, "The Means of Reproduction: Sex, Power, and the Future of the World" (Penguin Press, New York, 2009).

I discuss the exclusion of women from development economics in my book, *The Domestication of Women: discrimination in developing societies* (Tavistock, Methuen and Kogan Page, 1980). Since then there have been many initiatives to incorporate women's work and lives into development programmes. However these have often managed to avoid the issue covered here, so crucial to women, of being able to decide when or whether to have children.

Chapter nine

ACTIONS NOT WORDS
Turning the international debate
upside down

If we are to make modern contraception and safe terminations available to all who need them, we are at a turning point. We have the methods, the tried and tested programmes, and the experienced personnel. What we now need is a serious and consistent commitment from international and national contributors.

If people's basic need to control their own fertility is to be met, as an essential condition for economic development, then we all need to break out of our comfort zone, tear up some of the rule books, and challenge many of the International bodies and individual governments. Here are a few suggestions.

- The whole *economic development* movement should stop ignoring women's and families' need to make their own life decisions. They should understand the critical importance for anti-poverty moves of improving women's and families' welfare, as well as the need to avoid the catastrophe of environmental damage and runaway climate change. According to one estimate, the cost of meeting existing levels of demand for family planning in the United States and all developing countries ranges from US$3.6 billion to

US\$4.6 billion per year, which is just 5% of the annual global spending on climate change adaptation and the mitigation measures agreed in the Paris Agreement on Climate Change.

- *The IMF* should help to focus policy-makers' attention on the failure of governments to take this seriously, by dropping its simplistic GDP calculation for national income (which can be artificially inflated by more people) and moving to GDP per capita. This would more accurately show the state of an economy in terms of its people's real income, and highlight the economic benefit of family planning provision to enable people to stabilise the numbers. They should also attach an adequate value to a country's natural resources resulting from population growth, showing the loss of soils, water and wild areas in financial terms. As the environmentalist Sir David Attenborough commented, speaking of human numbers in 2013: "We have a finite environment – the planet. Anyone who thinks that you can have infinite growth in a finite environment is either a madman or an economist." The madmen may be a lost cause, but economists need to get on board now.

- The United Nations and its statisticians should stop using crude *dependency* calculations based on an arbitrary age kevel, and reflect the complexity of economically and socially active categories of the population which would show a much higher level of older people's contributions. This would demonstrate the levels of dependency created by inadequate health provision which creates high levels of illness and disability. The burden on women of unwanted pregnancies could also be highlighted in this way.

- *More research* is needed on the economic case for family planning as an element in poverty reduction programmes.

Deaths and injuries from unplanned pregnancies, and the negative effect on people's basic needs, should be valued as part of cost benefit analysis for development proposals. The real cost of supply failures, and illegal and dangerous abortion, should be fully understood in financial terms. Money talks, and this is especially true for economic development.

Health matters

- All *development and aid programmes,* whether for major infrastructure, formal education, agricultural development or whatever, should incorporate basic health services where these do not already exist, and supplement services where they do. This would provide an important confidence-building "quick win" element to the work, and also be of critical importance in its own right. The World Health Organisation (WHO) could draw up specifications for a minimum service to underpin all programmes and projects.

- *The World Health Organisation* needs to include family planning in all its field programmes, and member States could pursue this at WHO meetings. At the moment WHO does excellent work in research and drawing up guidelines for family planning, but it needs to go much further and demonstrate that it can integrate this fully into its practice.

- All health programmes should *include sexual and reproductive health* as an integral element. It should become unthinkable to offer health support without this. It is quite wrong, for example, that work should be done to prevent and treat *HIV/ AIDS* without offering reproductive health services, especially since anti-AIDS programmes have diverted some of the funds that would otherwise have gone to family planning. "Silo funding" or so-called "vertical programmes" can mean a gleaming modern building for AIDS and a shack with no facilities for maternity care next door. It reinforces a perception that women's lives simply do not matter.

• A particular issue arises with the public–private partnership, **The Global Fund** to Fight AIDS, Tuberculosis and Malaria, which raises and spends almost $4 billion a year. Targeting one disease out of context makes no sense if you neglect even the most basic health needs of the people, especially the women, who will remain very vulnerable to other indigenous diseases and future epidemics. Anti-AIDS work with no reproductive health element undermines people's trust in the programmes and ensures that more children have to face serious illness and disability.

• International health programmes, including the *"One Health"* movement, which currently focuses on links between zoonotic diseases passed from animals to humans, should widen their focus to include all human health issues including reproductive health. One Health is receiving very large amounts of funding from governments but currently seems to have little or no interest in human fertility. The funding should be conditional on their incorporating this crucial issue of health and welfare into all their work.

• Family planning projects are eligible for *climate change adaptation* funding, and international organisations and governments should incorporate family planning into their development plans. Adaptation to climate change is an important Sustainable Development Goal in its own right (SDG13) but many development organisations are likely to ignore this unless there is funding available.

• *Microfinance* organisations should recognise women's

need for small loans to pay for healthcare, including contraception, safe abortion and maternity care, which so often requires the payment of fees as well as the cost of travel to the nearest clinic or hospital. The local boards deciding on small loans should set up a small panel of health visitors, nurses, midwives or doctors, with no affiliation to anti-choice groups, who would be able to decide on people's requests for healthcare loans while guaranteeing their confidentiality. These panels should have their own loan fund and be able to decide quickly about the cases, which are often urgent. Not all health emergencies will be about pregnancy, but many will.

• Those of us who **give money** to international charities should stop and think about what their policies are. Why would I give to Oxfam or Unicef, for example, when they refuse to help women when they most need it? I will give to one of the family planning service groups that target this need. I do not claim that this will solve all problems everywhere, as critics like to pretend we are saying. But directing our small contributions this way helps to fill the yawning gap those "aid" organisations have created.

Ditch the conferences

• We should **switch the argument** from "rights" to "needs". The women's rights agenda, including freedom from sexual and other violence against women, will make better progress if it is not constantly challenged over "reproductive rights". Questions of child marriage, other forced marriage and FGM (female genital mutilation) should still be put forward as a human rights issue. The same applies to LGBTI (lesbian, gay, bisexual, transsexual and intersex). Human rights and particularly women's rights will move forward faster in this way. The reproductive health agenda will also work better if it is seen as a matter of basic needs and the fight against poverty.

- **The United Nations** should consider abandoning its format for conferences on women's rights and reproductive health since these have so often been sabotaged by the Holy See, alone or with a small number of delegations. Instead there should be consultations among all parties of good faith to draw up a *General Assembly resolution* on this. It would instruct all the specialised agencies – who are accountable to the General Assembly – to use their resources to support people's ability to make critical life decisions for themselves.

This resolution can be passed by a simple majority in the General Assembly, unlike the specialised conferences where absolute consensus has been required (for no obvious reason) and can be vetoed by the Holy See and a few others. A majority in the General Assembly should be easily achievable. A resolution along these lines could have a transformative effect for millions of people on the ground. There is a precedent for this in which I was involved: the General Assembly passed a resolution instructing the specialised agencies to prepare practical measures for the support of the former Portuguese colonies. They all swung into action, producing stamps, draft regulations and other elements for independent governments to hit the ground running once the Portuguese withdrew.

- The UN Fund for Population (UNFPA) could then become a *source of expertise and information* for all the agencies, and not just as the sole and insufficient source of operational funding.

Preparing for an unholy row

- *Permanent Representatives* of member States at the UN should challenge the status of the Holy See delegation, and its lack of any legal basis, and demand that it move to the same Observer status as other world religions. There has been silence on this for far too long.

- *Researchers in the field of international law* could usefully look into the status of the Holy See, to challenge its unauthorised access whether in the debates or behind the scenes, and recommend actions to stop its destructive tactics at the UN and at international conferences.

- *The Pope*, although he promised a "kinder and gentler" approach to human frailty rather than a condemnatory one, is not changing the dogmas on contraception and abortion. The hierarchy as a whole will – with differing degrees of severity – continue trying to persuade Catholics to follow the doctrine, until they can finally come to a more charitable view on this. However, they must recognise that they should not abuse their access to national and international forums to impose this on the vast majority of the world's people who are not Catholics or part of their "crusade". The Pope and the rest of the hierarchy should take a long, hard look at their diplomatic machine and its massive presence at international meetings, and cut it down to size. Persuasion is fine; coercion and manipulation are not. Their campaign against women's rights and especially family planning is damaging their presence in the international community.

- He should also stop *Catholic bishops'* pressure on those governments with largely Catholic populations. He should also issue firm guidelines to those church members who wish to oppose abortion or contraception, forbidding them to use any form of abuse, violence or threats of violence, whether against health personnel, patients or clinics. He should pull back the funding for front organisations and websites that are putting out misinformation. The Church's huge expenditure on international lobbying should be redirected to humanitarian assistance to all those in need, including so many millions of women and children who are suffering from unsupported childbirth, and from disasters, forced expulsions and war.

- Those claiming to speak in the name of **Islam and other major religions**, especially in international forums, also need to be challenged if they use them to pursue an agenda that follows that of the Holy See. If they are calling for more and more babies, they need to be confronted with the damage done to the needs of their people for good health, a family life they can sustain, and viable communities. Religious leaders should listen to their own people, especially the women, if they really want to improve their welfare. They should not try to impose their religious dogmas on members of other faiths, or none.

Filling the void

- The United States under Donald Trump is savagely cutting US contributions to international organisations, especially United Nations agencies dealing with family planning, climate change and the environment. **Other governments** around the world should urgently start to replace and increase this funding as a matter of urgency. While his "global gag" is in operation, seeking to silence any mention of pregnancy termination, they should adopt appropriate measures such as setting up separate organisations. They should also challenge the US Government in all international forums to stop trying to suppress non-US aid programmes.

- Since the United States, under Trump, may no longer be subscribing to much of the UN system, it will obviously be a painful *transition,* but it could set the UN and its agencies free to use their budgets to the fullest effect, free from US "gag" demands if US contributions have been stopped. It is estimated that a single dollar invested in family planning is worth six times that amount in other development areas, such as poverty reduction, education, or disaster preparedness projects. All donor countries should give much greater priority to this.

- *Developing nations'* governments will have to decide for themselves that health and family planning are a priority for their own budgets. Much has been done in many of these countries, with non-government organisations backed by national and international aid agencies, to introduce high-quality health programmes. However these can never reach the numbers of people needing them unless governments put their own resources into this. For many countries it will be difficult to meet the challenge, but it is essential if their people are to prosper. They should start by giving much greater support and encouragement to the *voluntary family planning organisations* in their own countries, which are already providing services, and encourage local government bodies, which often have their own budgets, to do the same.

- Public money could be withheld from *religious-based hospitals and clinics* if they do not offer a full range of reproductive health services. In more than a dozen countries in Africa, the "faith" sector is estimated at over

30% of all health services, often including district hospitals which oversee government facilities, and they usually operate by agreement with the government concerned. In the Democratic Republic of Congo it is over 50%. In areas where only Catholic clinics and hospitals exist, a separate family planning service could be set up – although it would be difficult to ensure that appropriate referrals would always be made. Alternatively, religious facilities can be incorporated into government health services, as has been done in South Africa. This obviously has to be done carefully, preserving the best of these facilities while incorporating vital family planning services. There could be a crucial role for the WHO in advising on a transition process.

• The *World Bank Group*, which is unexpectedly becoming a leader in developing integrated health finance and delivery, should bring together all other relevant UN agencies such as UNDP, WHO and Unicef, so that they can match their programmes with the Bank's, to improve universal health services to women and children. The same applies to the initiative "Every Woman Every Child", launched at UN headquarters by UN Secretary General Ban Ki-Moon in 2010, which aims to mobilise and intensify international and national action by governments, multilaterals, the private sector and non-governmental organisations. This office should be given greater powers and funding to achieve this.

Ending avoidance and evasion

• The *habit of avoidance* of this issue by some international civil servants needs to be continually challenged. For example, the United Nations resolutions on Women, Peace and Security specify reproductive health as an essential component of the security and status of women. Yet the UN global indicators on Women, Peace and Security that monitor the implementation of these resolutions, issued in 2016, do not include reproductive health indicators or guidelines. Such inconsistencies, the result of individual randomness, are unacceptable for such a critical issue.

• All those working in international agencies on the **Special Development Goals** and international aid programmes, including emergency relief and help for refugees, should also be required to include reproductive health. At the moment its inclusion is random and inconsistent. Writing about two high-level meetings on the same day on 19 September 2016, the United Nations General Assembly's High-Level Meeting on Refugees and Migrants, and US President Obama's Leaders' Summit on Refugees, Alison Doody of 2020 Vision writes: "The explicit inclusion of gender in high-level discussions is no longer remarkable, but remains inconsistent—sometimes taking priority, sometimes being mainstreamed into other issues, and at other times overlooked entirely. The situation is even starker, however, when it comes to sexual and reproductive health, which is too often still not given the priority of a life-saving intervention. This means SRH care can make it into one part of a declaration on refugees, but is entirely absent from another summit the same week."

• Another void is *food security:* women and girls make up the majority of food-insecure people globally, and unwanted pregnancies add greatly to this burden. Yet it was omitted from the conversation on World Food Day of the same year.

• Those who indulge in censorship of the issues should be *challenged* and, if necessary, disciplined. It is a matter for the Secretary General of the UN and the heads of all the UN agencies. The UN's Every Woman, Every Child office could be the best placed to monitor this and report to the Secretary General for action.

Leaving the comfort zone

• *Family planning organisations,* whether national or international ones, should stop being defensive and even secretive and start communicating widely about what they are doing. At the moment they are mainly preaching to the converted in terms of modern contraceptive and early abortion methods, and how these are best offered in different situations. I would hope to see open seminars and conferences on a range of relevant topics, open to the whole development "Establishment": aid officials, women's and environmental groups and development academics.

• *Show what* you are doing, *how and why.* Tackle the ignorance of modern methods and the misinformation and prejudice that lingers from Germaine Greer's misinformed *Sex and Destiny* and is being spread around by the opposition, such as imagined coercion or malpractice and wildly exaggerated claims about side effects from contraceptives. Hire security for your meetings if you are worried about the lynch mob. A bit less jargon would also be welcome, with a real effort to speak the language of ordinary people and a clearout of all the abbreviations and jargon.

• *The media* at all levels – local, national and international – should regularly report on health and family planning initiatives, and their successes. Too much "news" in this area is negative, focusing only on fundamentalist opposition: otherwise it ignores these critical issues completely. There is a clear parallel with media coverage of climate change: too little, too conflicted, too late.

- The whole international system should adopt the *mission statement* of the UNFPA: "Delivering a world where every pregnancy is wanted, every childbirth is safe and every young person's potential is fulfilled." Or, to use another family planning slogan: "Every child a wanted child." The people of the world, and future generations, depend on it.

A BRIEF BIBLIOGRAPHY

I have done extensive searches and found almost no books that address the "population" issue as one of women in development, or any that focus on the issue of individual decisions about children as key to overall population numbers. There is an avoidance of women's choices as key to this, perhaps because almost all the authors are men. The outstanding exception to this is Michelle Goldberg's *The Means of Reproduction: sex, power and the future of the world (Penguin, New York, 2009)* which examines the US and global battles over women's reproductive rights, and is mainly reportage. It does not examine successful programmes in detail or offer specific ways forward, which is what I have tried to do. Robert Engelman of the WorldWatch Institute has also raised the issue of women being central to population issues, as "a first word not a last word," in *More: Population, Nature, and What Women Want* (Island Press, Washington DC, 2008).

The most influential recent book on the other side, especially in Europe, is probably Danny Dorling's book *Population 10 Billion (Constable, 2013)*. However he fails to discuss in any detail the question of preventing unwanted pregnancy, nor is there any reference to this being a women's issue. His references to contraception in general are dismissive. His conclusion – that something could turn up to solve the problem of human population growth – is complacent and in serious need of challenge.

There have been a number of often alarmist books that warn of the dangers of rapidly increasing population, including Paul Ehrlich's *The Population Bomb* (Buccaneer, 1968, 1971), and Stephen Emmott's *10 Billion*. The titles show that they are looking at the numbers, not the individuals behind the numbers. Their failure to discuss individual experience, or even of contraception as an issue, leaves all their warnings at a level of abstract policy which is unlikely to be heeded, and could even feed into the accusation that this is about "population control" even though that is not their intention.

Lester R Brown has published a series of useful books including *Full Planet, Empty Plates* (Norton, 2012) and (with Hal Kane) *Full House* (Earthscan, 1995). Fred Pearce's *Peoplequake* and Thomas L Friedman's *Hot, Flat, and Crowded* (Penguin, 2009) are similar. These and other such books, including several by Robert Engelman, are attempting to position this as a key environmental issue. However the green movement as a whole has been very resistant and is now only just beginning to see the connections with family planning.

There is a specialist area of contraception and family planning studies (but not in book form), which offers a wealth of information, especially on the increasingly successful approaches to choice, which are showing great success though held back by a lack of funding. This is very much preaching to the converted and is little known in the development and environmental worlds. I aim to provide an essential information link to the development arena to show what can and should be done.

A critical element in this debate is what I am calling the New Eugenics – an alliance of fundamentalists, right-wingers, the Catholic Church hierarchy and various "right to life" groups. There are several influential pro-natalist books focused on race, with apocalyptic titles like Jonathan V Last's *What to Expect When No-one's Expecting* (Encounter Books, 2013), Mark Steyn's *America Alone: The End of the World as we Know it* (Regnery Press, 2006), or Pat Buchanan's *The Death of the West: How Dying Populations and Immigrant Invasions imperil our Country and* Civilisation *(St Martin's Press, 2001)*, and several others.

OTHER PUBLICATIONS BY BARBARA ROGERS

The Domestication of Women: discrimination in developing societies (Tavistock, Methuen and Kogan Page, 1980) is credited with boosting the integration of women into the international development process. Extensively reviewed, invitations to speak at international conferences. This book became a standard academic text and influenced the integration of women in international development.

> "A cogent manifesto to which the scholarship of anthropology, economics, statistics,
> and development studies is convincingly harnessed."
> (*New Society)*

Men Only: An investigation into men's organisations (Pandora, 1988) tackled male networking and argued successfully for the abolition of public subsidies to men-only areas at private clubs in the UK, including Lord's cricket ground.

> "One always has a certain admiration for those who try to research primitive tribes, so I took my hat off this week to the doughty Ms Barbara Rogers … who set out to investigate the world of men's clubs."
> (*Sunday Times)*

52%: getting women's power into politics (Women's Press, 1983) was the first book to look at a whole range of policy issues, and women's importance as swing voters. Extracts published in *Woman* entitled "So this is liberation".

> "This is her vivid and controversial polemic, arguing that women must realise that traditional politics are too important to leave alone." (*Time Out*)

Divide and Rule: South Africa's Bantustans (International Defence and Aid, various editions) informed international decision-making on whether to recognise South Africa's puppet regimes, and contributed to the failure of this key *apartheid* policy.

The Nuclear Axis (JF Publishing and Times Books, 1978) exposed South Africa's secret nuclear weapons programme under the *apartheid* regime. South Africa is now the first country in the world to dismantle its nuclear weapons.

White Wealth and Black Poverty: American Investments in Southern Africa (Greenwood Press, 1976*)* helped to kick-start the movement to disinvest in *apartheid* South Africa.

> 'Rogers' forceful case for U.S. economic disengagement from South Africa is buttressed by a detailed description of the parallel development of apartheid and industrialization in South Africa ... this study provides a valuable resource, superseding in breadth and depth most current analyses of the subject." *(Foreign Affairs)*

Race: No peace without justice (World Council of Churches, 1980) is the result of extensive consultation among churches around the world, and has been used as an educational text since then.

Barbara Rogers has also produced research and analysis on Africa, international development and women's issues for the United Nations, UNDP and FAO, the Chair of the US House of Representatives Africa Subcommittee, Anti-Slavery International, Change and various charities. She was the founding Editor of the current affairs magazine *Everywoman* where she worked for nine years. Her books are written to influence national and international policy, aiming to recast international issues in accessible terms to influence academic debate, but also to reach beyond it to reach opinion formers on issues that are of crucial importance to us all.